AAC and Aided Language in the Classroom

Have you got learners in your class who have Speech, Language, and Communication Needs (SLCN) who would benefit from resources to support their communication skills, such as using Aided Language/Augmentative and Alternative Communication (AAC)?

This empowering book is designed with these questions at its heart. Written in an accessible style, by teachers for teachers, it offers guidance and support to help you to overcome barriers and successfully implement AAC. The book:

- Addresses myths and misconceptions, with discussion points to encourage the reader to reflect on their own practice.
- Shares the current evidence base around successful support strategies.
- Includes easy to implement, practical strategies that can be adopted in any classroom to have maximum impact and enhance learners' communication skills.
- Contains a wealth of relatable, real-life examples and case studies included throughout, to bring theory to life and help you deliver effective classroom practice and support your learners with SLCN.
- Clearly outlines the variety of different assistive technologies available for facilitating communication.

Providing readers with a range of useful tools and resources to implement Aided Language/AAC, *AAC and Aided Language in the Classroom* builds practitioners' confidence and enables educators to provide a universal level of support for learners with SLCN. It is valuable reading for school leaders, SENCOs, teachers, and learning support assistants, as well as speech and language therapists supporting educators with the implementation of Aided Language/AAC.

Katy Leckenby is a Senior AAC Consultant for Ace Centre, a national charity providing support and advice to people with complex needs around the use of Assistive Technology (ATech) and Augmentative and Alternative Communication (AAC). Katy is passionate about facilitating communication and removing barriers to ensure that all students can fully access education. She holds an MA in Inclusive Education and was a teacher for seventeen years, starting in Primary then moving into Special Education, where she taught young people with ASC, MLD, SLD, PMLD and complex needs.

Meaghan Ebbage-Taylor is a Senior AAC Consultant for Ace Centre and a trained Primary School teacher. She has worked within a special school, teaching pupils with a range of communication difficulties, including those who have made use of a wide range of AAC, both paper-based and electronic. Meaghan's teaching background has given her a good insight into the everyday implementation of AAC within a classroom context and how to support this to meet the communication need of individuals to get their voice heard.

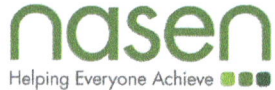

NASEN is a professional membership association that supports all those who work with or care for children and young people with special and additional educational needs. Members include SENCOs, school leaders, governors/trustees, teachers, teaching assistants, support workers, other educationalists, students and families.

NASEN supports its members through policy documents, peer-reviewed academic journals, its membership magazine, *nasen Connect*, publications, professional development courses, regional networks and newsletters. Its website contains more current information, such as responses to government consultations.

NASEN'S published documents are held in very high regard, both in the UK and internationally.

For a full list of titles see: www.routledge.com/nasen-spotlight/book-series/FULNASEN

Other titles published in association with the National Association for Special Educational Needs (NASEN):

AAC and Aided Language in the Classroom: Breaking Down Barriers for Learners with Speech, Language and Communication Needs
Katy Leckenby and Meaghan Ebbage-Taylor
2025/pb: 978-1-032-53196-0

Supporting Children and Young People Through Loss and Trauma: Hands-On Strategies to Improve Wellbeing and Mental Health
Juliet Taylor
2024/pb: 978-1-032-23023-8

Language for Learning in the Primary School: A Practical Guide for Supporting Pupils with Language and Communication Difficulties across the Curriculum, 3rd ed.
Sue Hayden and Emma Jordan
2023/pb: 978-1-032-34259-7

Beating Bureaucracy in Special Educational Needs: Helping SENCOs Maintain a Work/Life Balance, 4th ed
Jean Gross
2023/pb: 978-1-032-32239-1

Inclusive and Accessible Science for Students with Additional or Special Needs: How to Teach Science Effectively to Diverse Learners in Secondary Schools
Jane Essex
2023/pb: 978-0-367-76627-6

True Partnerships in SEND: Working Together to Give Children, Families and Professionals a Voice
Heather Green and Becky Edwards
2023/pb: 978-0-367-54494-2

Teaching Reading to All Learners Including those with Complex Needs
Sarah Moseley
2023/pb: 978-1-032-11475-0

AAC and Aided Language in the Classroom
Breaking Down Barriers for Learners with Speech, Language and Communication Needs

Katy Leckenby and Meaghan Ebbage-Taylor

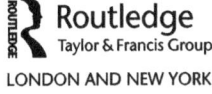

LONDON AND NEW YORK

Designed cover image: Meaghan Ebbage Taylor

First published 2025
by Routledge
4 Park Square, Milton Park, Abingdon, Oxon OX14 4RN

and by Routledge
605 Third Avenue, New York, NY 10158

Routledge is an imprint of the Taylor & Francis Group, an informa business

© 2025 Katy Leckenby and Meaghan Ebbage-Taylor

The right of Katy Leckenby and Meaghan Ebbage-Taylor to be identified as authors of this work has been asserted in accordance with sections 77 and 78 of the Copyright, Designs and Patents Act 1988.

All rights reserved. The purchase of this copyright material confers the right on the purchasing institution to photocopy or download pages which bear the support material icon and a copyright line at the bottom of the page. No other parts of this book may be reprinted or reproduced or utilised in any form or by any electronic, mechanical, or other means, now known or hereafter invented, including photocopying and recording, or in any information storage or retrieval system, without permission in writing from the publishers.

Trademark notice: Product or corporate names may be trademarks or registered trademarks, and are used only for identification and explanation without intent to infringe.

British Library Cataloguing-in-Publication Data
A catalogue record for this book is available from the British Library

ISBN: 9781032531953 (hbk)
ISBN: 9781032531960 (pbk)
ISBN: 9781003410836 (ebk)

DOI: 10.4324/9781003410836

Typeset in Helvetica Neue LT Std
by Newgen Publishing UK

Access the Support Material: resourcecentre.routledge.com/books/9781032531960

Contents

Preface	vii
1 More Than the Freedom of Speech	1
2 Lifting the Veil of Terminology	9
3 Myths and Misconceptions: What the Research Tells Us	19
4 Education Is Not an Island: The Importance of Teamwork	27
5 What We Already Know	37
6 Getting the Environment Right	45
7 What is Symbolic Language?	59
8 How Do We Teach Symbolic Language?	65
9 Modelling	77
10 Language Development: The Danger Zone of Just Requesting	91
11 Low Cost, Effective Resources	103
12 Communication Partner Skills	119
13 Supporting Access to Aided Language for Learners with Physical Disabilities	137
14 Assessment and Target Setting	163
15 Opportunities: Pupil Voice	173
16 Whole School Approach to Supporting Learners with Speech, Language and Communication Needs	181
17 Final Thoughts	189
Index	191

Preface

We are experienced teachers and currently work as AAC Consultants at the national charity Ace Centre, who work with people of all ages who use or need Augmentative and Alternative Communication (AAC) and Assistive Technology (ATech) to communicate. We have experienced first-hand the lack of initial teacher training and the national shortage of speech and language therapy support, around how to teach learners with Speech, Language and Communication Needs (SLCN). When teaching we were able to identify learners who had a need for support but felt helpless in how to break down those communication barriers. This was due to the lack of training and information available around effective classroom practice using aided language/AAC. Skill development came via any opportunities provided by specialist organisations, such as Ace Centre or taster opportunities from suppliers of Augmentative and Alternative Communication systems, in a try-before-you-buy manner and online webinars.

Unlike other publications in this area, this book covers the topic of aided language/AAC in the classroom from the perspective of teachers who have worked within the education system in England and understand the current Department for Education (DfE) guidance.

The book offers useful advice and signposts to a range of resources to get you started with your journey of implementing aided language/AAC into your classrooms for learners with Speech, Language and Communication Needs.

Remember, aided language is not just for curriculum answers – autonomous communication is the ultimate goal!

Access Your Online Resources

AAC and Aided Language in the Classroom is accompanied by a number of printable online materials, designed to ensure this resource best supports your professional needs.

Go to resourcecentre.routledge.com/books/9781032531960 and answer the question prompt, using your copy of the book to gain access to the online content.

1 More Than the Freedom of Speech

As teachers we feel the deepest commitment to enabling all of our learners to achieve their full potential. This is even more pronounced when we meet a learner with speech, language and communication needs (SLCN). Freedom of speech is a basic human right protected by the Human Rights Act 1998, Article 10 Freedom of Expression, but as Stephen Hawking once said, 'More important than the freedom of speech is the freedom to speak.'

The goal for all our learners is that they leave education equipped to actively participate in society to live full and enriched lives. There is a need to be able to share thoughts and feelings, communicate choices about various aspects of life and engage in a way that fosters relationships with others. Sharing language is the basis of communication which facilitates those interactions. If a learner does not have access to language to express themselves, they are likely to experience many communication breakdowns which can lead to frustration, withdrawal, or even worse, learned helplessness. Many students who do not have access to that shared language will rely on others to interpret behaviours, which may lead to problematic behaviour when communicating negative emotions. An example of this may be a learner pushing someone when they do not have the expressive language to ask or tell that person to 'go'.

Has there been a time in your life when you were unable to communicate verbally? Did you rely on alternative communication, writing notes or sending digital messages, such as e-mail or text? When you could not use your verbal expressive language, did that mean you did not generate language in your head? The answer is yes, of course you still generate language in your head, even if you do not have the means to communicate and share it with another person at that time. It is clear that we have our inner voice, no matter if we can't say it out loud and for the majority of students that we come across, with Speech language and communication needs, this will also be the case. How much language and the complexity of that language will depend on the learner's level of cognition. This is irrespective of a learner's ability to convey their thoughts and feelings.

Vygotsky, 1986, highlighted how the inner voice develops as early as age three, so imagine generating all of that internal speech and not being able to share it. It's no wonder that learners with significant speech, language and communication needs display frustration around the lack of means to express themselves.

With mental health being at the forefront of educator's minds following the COVID 19 pandemic, where people experienced being isolated from society. It is key that we acknowledge the importance of being able to communicate with others to express ourselves for good mental health. We also need to acknowledge the impact that lack of expressive communication can have on learners with significant speech language and communication needs. The Royal College of Speech and Language Therapists Clinical Information on Mental Health (adults) 2023 highlights that 'People with a primary communication difficulty are at a greater risk of experiencing mental health problems than their peers, commonly anxiety and depression.'

With this in mind it is clear to see why legislation is in place to ensure that all learners should have a voice, even if they are not using verbal communication, and that their voice is heard and given due weight. In the education sector this is often referred to as gaining pupil voice but, to strip that back to its most basic form, we are talking about communication and social participation. Giving learners the means to be able to express themselves and actively participate in their own lives.

School settings may have policy to promote gaining pupil voice and also a communication policy to outline how the needs of learners with speech, language and communication needs will be met. These policies will often use terms such as *Total Communication* and will give examples of strategies which may be used to support learners. However, unlike many of the other policies within a school setting, it is worthwhile to note that there is legislation around supporting communication for learners. Hindering support in this area, however unintentional, could lead to this legislation being enforced against the school. Therefore, you could liken the communication policy to policies such as the health and safety policy, rather than a curriculum subject. Writing an AAC policy features in a later chapter and encourages the inclusion of the legislation detailed below.

> The United Nations (UN) Convention on the Rights of Persons with Disabilities (CRPD) Article 24 – Education provides the clearest guidance on the legal requirements of schools.
>
> 3. States Parties shall enable persons with disabilities to learn life and social development skills to facilitate their full and equal participation in education and as members of the community. To this end, States Parties shall take appropriate measures, including:
>
>   a) Facilitating the learning of Braille, alternative script, augmentative and alternative modes, means and formats of communication and orientation and mobility skills, and facilitating peer support and mentoring;
>   b) Facilitating the learning of sign language and the promotion of the linguistic identity of the deaf community;
>   c) Ensuring that the education of persons, and in particular children, who are blind, deaf or deafblind, is delivered in the most appropriate languages and modes and means of communication for the individual, and in environments which maximize academic and social development.

Initial teacher training rarely teaches that there is legislation which states that a child with complex communication needs should be facilitated to learn alternative modes of communication, such as alternative, augmentative communication (AAC). This places the responsibility on everyone who is supporting the learner. Not just at the feet of a speech and language therapist. Implementation of AAC to support a learner's communication, is the responsibility of everyone.

This theme continues with The United Nations Convention on the Rights of the Child 1989 (Articles 12 and 13):

> Children have a right to receive and impart information, to express an opinion and to have that opinion taken into account in any matters affecting them from the early years. Their views should be given due weight according to their age, maturity and capability.

Case Example

This is an example of a learner who has speech, language and communication needs, who uses the alternative mode of a communication book to support his expressive language. Marcin was chatting with his teacher Carly about what he wants to do when he leaves his specialist school. This was in preparation of information to be shared as part of his Educational Health Care Plan review meeting. Using his paper-based communication book, Marcin told his teacher that he wanted to drive a police car and be Father Christmas. With Marcin being fifteen years old, there is a danger that educators would want to say that was not a valid answer, and that he needed to choose something else. Thankfully, Carly did not do that. Instead, she entered into a conversation with him about what he would do if he became Father Christmas. This was the teacher meeting the learner at his level, giving *due weight to his communication according to his age, maturity and capability*. If a young verbal child came to us and told us that they were going to be Spider Man, we would not correct them. Instead, we would talk about Spider Man and they would express their thoughts and feelings on the topic and all of that expressive language shared would be valued (Figure 1.1).

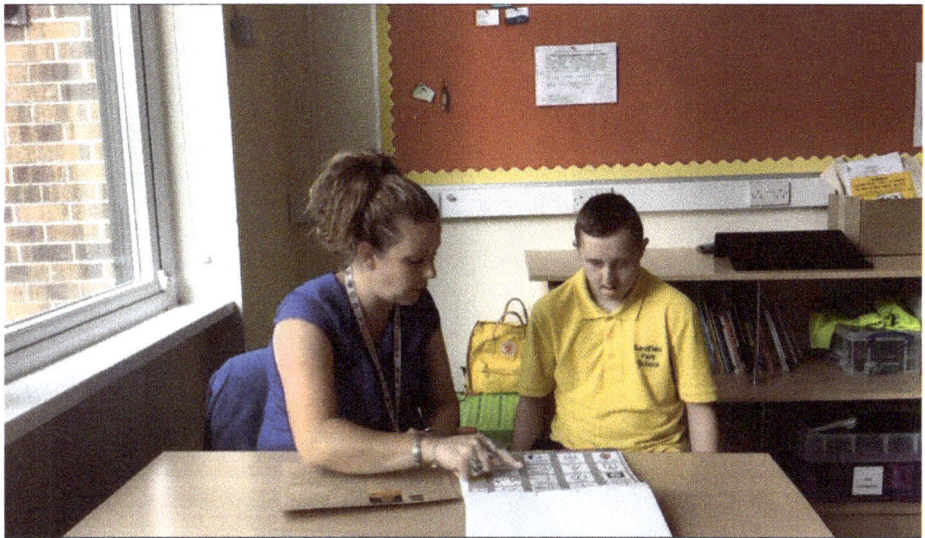

Figure 1.1 A woman and a teenage boy using a PODD communication book.

Source: Photographed for author by Carly Hinds.

Discussion Point!

Now picture that non-verbal learner or learner who has unintelligible speech in your classroom.
- How would that currently play out for them if they had to share their hopes and aspirations for the future?
- Do they have access to expressive language, or would they need an alternative mode of communication to support them to share their dreams and aspirations like Marcin?
- When we are thinking about communication in the classroom, it is clear to see that we are legally bound to facilitate learners to 'impart information and to express an opinion'.

SEND Code of Practice

In 2001, the SEN Code of Practice proposed the concept of 'pupil participation' this consolidated the idea of Pupil Voice in education. 'The right of children with special educational needs to be involved in making decisions and exercising choices.' The legislation highlights the importance of the learner's 'voice' being heard and the need for the learner to participate in decisions about their own lives, ready to take their place in society. The SEN Code of Practice set clear guidelines that the local authority must provide the opportunity for the learner to share 'views, wishes and feelings ... participating as fully as possible in decisions, and being provided with the information and support necessary to enable participation in those discussions.'

In 2014 England saw the introduction of Education Health and Care Plans, EHCPs, with the aim of joining up the education, health and care services to offer a child centred approach to supporting the learner, with their needs being at the forefront. The EHCPs cover four broad areas with communication being one of those to highlight the importance of being able to communicate as a basic human right. This advocated that services and support should work collaboratively to meet the learner's needs.

The Revised SEN Code of practice (2015) echoed the 2001 SEN Code of practice, reiterating pupil participation in decision making by involving them in discussions and actively supporting them to 'contributing to needs assessments, developing and reviewing Education, Health and Care Plans (EHCPs)'.

> The SEND review 2022: Right Support, Right Place, Right Time, continues to confirm that the young person's voice should be central in decisions about their education and life. It outlined the introduction of consistent standards for *'co-production and communication with children, young people and their families so that they are engaged in the decision-making process around the support that they receive and the progress they are making.'*

The danger is that, although these legislations should ensure that pupil voice is central in any educational processes, the professional rhetoric is rarely transferred into actual practice where the learner is able to express their thoughts and feelings. Rather, learners are advocated for by adults who know them. Imagine what it would be like if a close friend or partner was the one who expressed your views on your life to others: could they ever know every thought in your head? The answer is of course 'no', and that is why we must find appropriate ways for learners to communicate their own thoughts and feelings. Then nothing is lost in translation. Learners will then be able to have autonomy over their lives and have control over matters that affect them, rather than being helpless in getting their thoughts and feelings heard and understood.

Some schools have adopted using a Communication Bill of Rights as a clear visual to represent what responsibilities the school staff hold in regard to facilitating the effective communication of their learners. Here is an image of James Rennie School's Communication Bill of Rights (Figure 1.2), which is displayed on the wall in their school in Carlisle.

Having a visual display such as this is an effective way to remind all staff and visitors to the school of the rights of the learners. Other schools, such as Green Fold Special School in Bolton, have opted to use a visual of the Communication Bill of Rights in their Communication Policy (Figure 1.3), as they felt that a visual clearly communicated the rights of their learners, and did this in an accessible way for all learners, staff, and family members and other visitors.

The SEND review green paper in 2022 informed that since 2015, there has been an increase in the proportion of children and young people with EHCPs, with a primary need of speech, language and communication needs and, amongst pupils on SEN Support in state-funded primary schools, the most common primary need in 2021 was speech, language and communication needs (34%).

Once a learner is identified as having speech, language and communication needs and is waiting for speech and language therapy intervention, there can often be a general acceptance

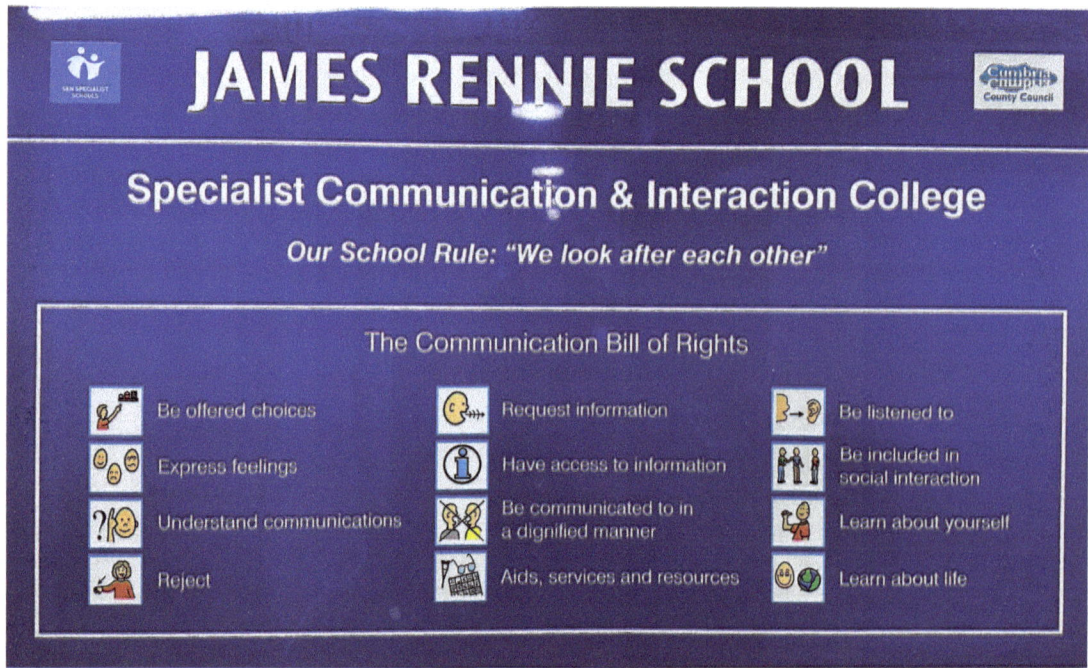

Figure 1.2 A display board labelled James Rennie School.

Source: Photographed by the author.

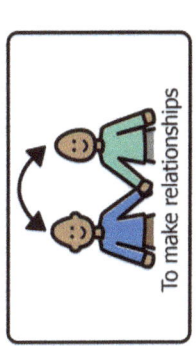
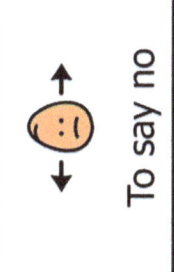
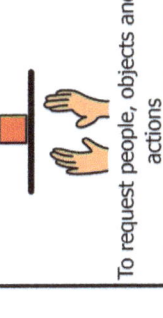
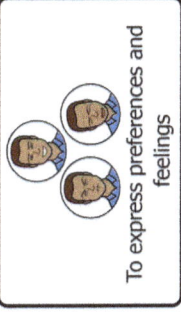
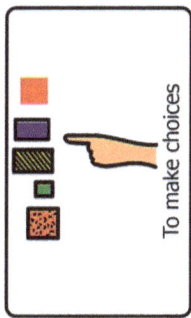
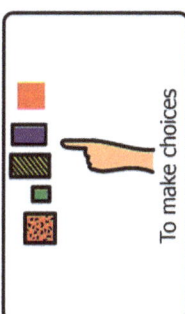
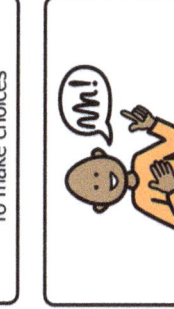
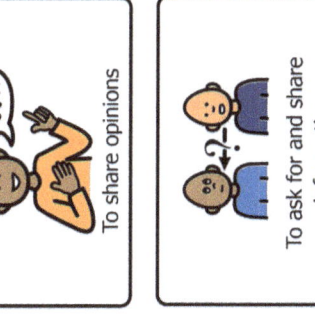
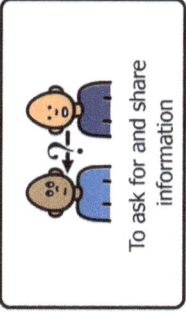
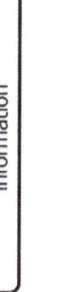
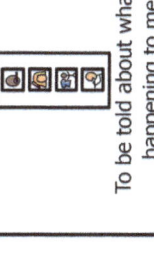
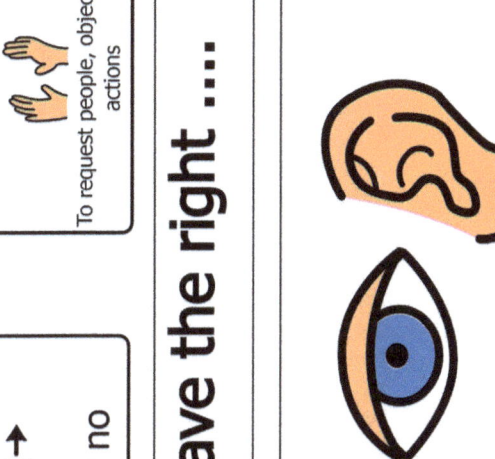
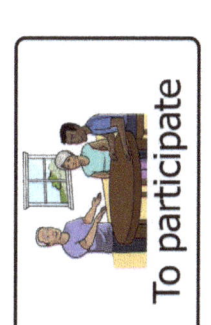
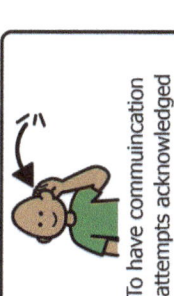
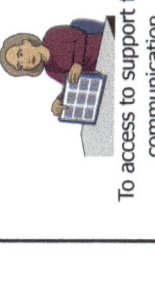
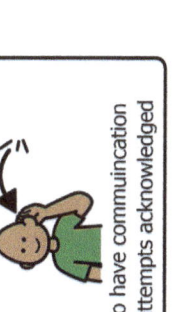
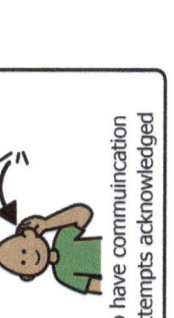
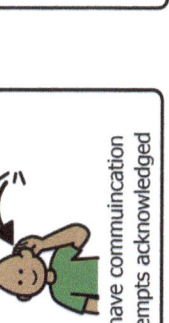
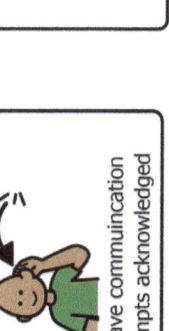
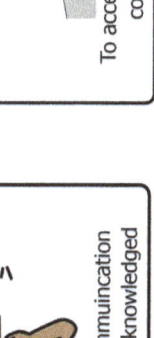

Figure 1.3 A symbol picture board titled 'I have the right'.

Source: Created by the author using PCS symbols. PCS and Boardmaker are trademarks of Tobii Dynavox LLC. All rights reserved. Used with permission.

Copyright material from Katy Leckenby and Meaghan Ebbage-Taylor (2025), *AAC and Aided Language in the Classroom* Routledge

of passing responsibility for the rights of that child around their communication needs onto the speech and language therapist – with educators feeling they do not have the skills, knowledge and understanding in order to meet these learner's communication needs.

There is often an expectation that the learner's communication need will be 'fixed' by the therapist and educators, and that those around the learner do not have a part to play. This view links closely to the medical model of disability, where there is an emphasis on the person needing to be 'fixed' to be able to function within society. The reality of the situation is likely that there may be a long waiting period for the learner to be seen by a therapist, and the therapy will be a process which will have a much higher success rate if strategies and support are used all day everyday with all communication partners, not just within the designated therapy time.

Whilst waiting for interventions to be put in place to support learners, and once these begin, we as educators need to be mindful that support for learners to effectively express themselves still happens. Therefore, we must look at the social model of disability and meet the learner where they are and look at what can be adapted to assist them to fully participate in their education. This could be likened to a child waiting to receive glasses as they have a visual impairment. The learner would not be left at the back of the class until they received their glasses. Instead, class staff would seek out strategies which may somewhat compensate until the child receives their glasses, such as offering them a place nearer to the information being shared on the board or pairing them with someone who could read the information that they could not see themselves. This is the same for a learner who is waiting for a speech and language therapy assessment. Educators must make alterations to teaching to make participation accessible.

This book explores how educators can support those learners for whom verbal speech is not a reliable option, either due to lack of clarity or an absence of verbal speech altogether.

It is worth noting that this book is not to replace the skills of a speech and language therapist, but rather to support educators in ensuring that the rights of a child can be met.

A report from the Children's Commissioner for England in June 2019 'showed a real terms reduction in spending on children's Speech and Language Therapy (SLT) in the majority of areas in England between 2016 and 2019'. It went on to highlight that, 'although total SLT spend in England rose from £143m in 2016–17 to £166m in 2018–19, most areas (57%) saw a real terms decrease in spending on services to improve children's communication skills.' Access to support from NHS speech and language therapy for learners with speech, language and communication needs is also being impacted by a general decline in professionals working at that specialist level. This can often result in teaching staff identifying that there is a need for intervention but feeling left in the dark on how to offer the most basic support whilst waiting for speech and language therapy input.

Conclusion

In this chapter we have looked at how key legislation and the SEND Code of Practice raise awareness of the responsibilities of educators to use support tools such as aided language in the classroom environment.

The following chapters of the book look at general support strategies, which cover some of the basic groundwork that can be done within the classroom environment to support learners with speech, language and communication needs, some of whom may be waiting for assessment or intervention with a speech and language therapist, and some who have not yet been referred. One thing is certain though: Just because a child cannot speak, it does not mean that the child has nothing say.

Bibliography

Children's Commissioner for England (2019). Lack of Funding for Children's Speech and Language Therapy. Available at: www.publicfinance.co.uk/news/2019/06/lack-funding-childrens-speech-and-language-therapy

Department for Education (2001). Special Educational Needs Code of Practice. Ref: DfES/581/2001. Available at: www.gov.uk/government/publications/special-educational-needs-sen-code-of-practice

Department for Education and Department of Health (2015). Special Educational Needs and Disability Code of Practice: 0 to 25 years. Ref: DFE-00205-2013 Available at: www.gov.uk/government/publications/send-code-of-practice-0-to-25

Department for Education and Department of Health (2022). SEND Review: Right support Right place Right time. Available at: https://assets.publishing.service.gov.uk/media/624178c68fa8f5277c0168e7/SEND_review_right_support_right_place_right_time_accessible.pdf

The Royal College of Speech and Language Therapists (2023). Clinical Information on Mental Health (adults). Available at: www.rcslt.org/speech-and-language-therapy/clinical-information/mental-health-adults/#:~:text=There%20are%20important%20links%20between%20mental%20health%20and,mental%20health%20problems%20may%20also%20have%20communication%20needs

The United Nations Convention on the Rights of the Child (1989). Articles 12 and 13.

The United Nations (UN) Convention on the Rights of Persons with Disabilities (CRPD) Article 24.

Vygotsky, L.S. (1986). *Thought and language*. Cambridge, Mass.: MIT Press.

2 Lifting the Veil of Terminology

As with many areas of education, it is easy to become tied down by the countless number of acronyms and complex terminology used without clear explanation. This can cause confusion and misconceptions, which leads to barriers to successful implementation.

This chapter will explain terminology relating to Speech, Language and Communication Needs (SLCN), Augmentative and Alternative Communication (AAC) and aided language. This will break down those barriers relating to the specialist jargon in a user-friendly way to stop educators becoming overwhelmed.

Learners with Speech Language and Communication Needs (are often identified by educators as presenting with Special Educational Needs and Disabilities (SEND) under the SEND Code of Practice (2015), which is split into 4 key areas:

- Cognition and Learning – learners with specific learning difficulties, a moderate, severe or profound and multiple learning disability.
- Communication and Interaction – learners with Speech Language and Communication Needs (SLCN), which includes autistic learners and learners with complex communication needs whose verbal speech is not sufficient to meet their daily needs.
- Social, Emotional and Mental Health – learners with emotional, social and mental health difficulties.
- Sensory and/or physical difficulties – learners with visual, hearing or multi-sensory impairment and physical disabilities.

This book focusses on learners identified as having SLCN. It may be useful here to think about what is meant by Speech Language and Communication Needs.

The Royal College of Speech and Language Therapists (2009) set these out as follows:

- problems with producing speech sounds accurately
- stammering
- voice problems, such as hoarseness and loss of voice
- problems understanding language (making sense of what people say)
- problems using language (words and sentences)
- problems interacting with others. For example, difficulties understanding the non-verbal rules of good communication or using language in different ways to question, clarify or describe things.

Learners with Speech Language and Communication Needs may have receptive or expressive language difficulties, or difficulties in both areas.

A receptive language difficulty causes learners to struggle to understand language. Whereas an expressive language difficulty causes a learner to struggle expressing thoughts, wants and needs, predominantly through speech.

Learners identified as having receptive or expressive language difficulties often benefit from a *total communication environment*. This is a term which is used by many schools, but it may be useful here to unpick this term a little to make sure we are clear what this means. Some examples of multimodal communication are included below:

- Speech
- Body language
- Gesture
- Pointing, looking and showing
- Alternative and Augmentative Communication (AAC)

DOI: 10.4324/9781003410836-2

But what is Alternative and Augmentative Communication (AAC)? This is an umbrella term, covering strategies to either support and supplement or replace speech. The International Society for Augmentative and Alternative Communication (2011) outlines AAC as, "a set of tools and strategies that an individual uses to solve every day communicative challenges".

> **Discussion Point!**
>
> - What type of learners do you have within your classroom?
> - Would their Speech Language and communication needs fit into any of the above?
> - What tools do you currently have in place to support them?

AAC can be Characterised as either Unaided or Aided

Unaided Communication does not involve the use of equipment, such as speaking, gesturing or signing.

Aided Communication involves the use of additional equipment, such as communication charts, communication books, or a communication aid. This book will focus on the implementation of aided language in the classroom.

AAC can be text to speech, where messages are typed and then spoken out for individuals who are literate. This book will solely focus on the use of symbol based AAC for learners who are still developing their literacy skills.

A symbol is anything that is used to represent something else e.g., a cup for a drink, a photograph of a dog or symbol on a high-tech communication system.

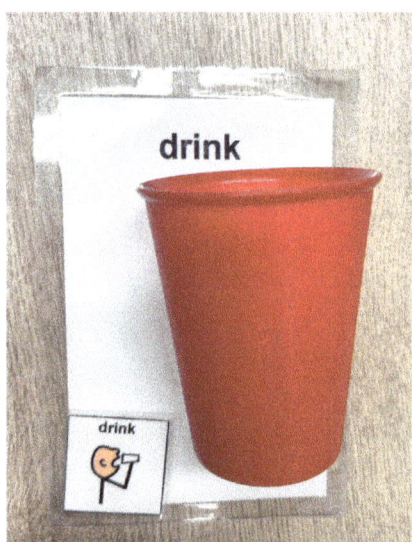

Figure 2.1 A red cup with the word *drink*.
Source: Photographed by the author.

Examples of AAC that are Commonly used in Schools

Objects of reference (Figure 2.1): Use of real objects to represent an activity, for example a seatbelt to represent going on the bus, or a plate and cup to represent snack time. This image shows a picture of a spoon to represent lunch.

Paper-based strategies are frequently used, which are not reliant on power. These include the use of writing, photographs, drawings and graphic symbols. Next are some examples of different paper-based resources.

Picture Communication System (PECS) (Figure 2.2), which is a structured approach, with six stages, to develop communication, allowing a learner with limited language to communicate through photos or symbols. At the beginning stages the learner gives a picture of a desired item in exchange for the corresponding item. These early stages teach how to request and ask for given items. This focusses heavily on teaching learners to initiate interactions with a communication partner, rather than focusing on language development. This is based on ABA applied behavioural analysis, which primarily focusses on behavioural change.

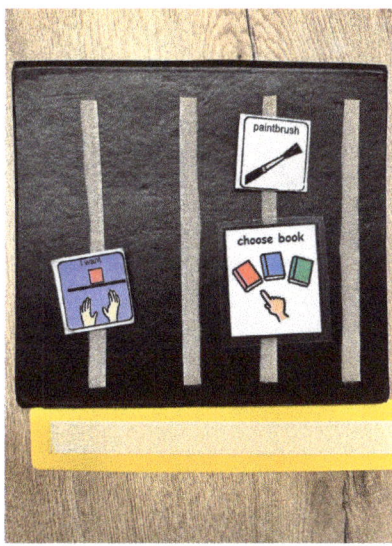

Figure 2.2 A black folder with three symbols on the top.

Source: Photographed by the author.

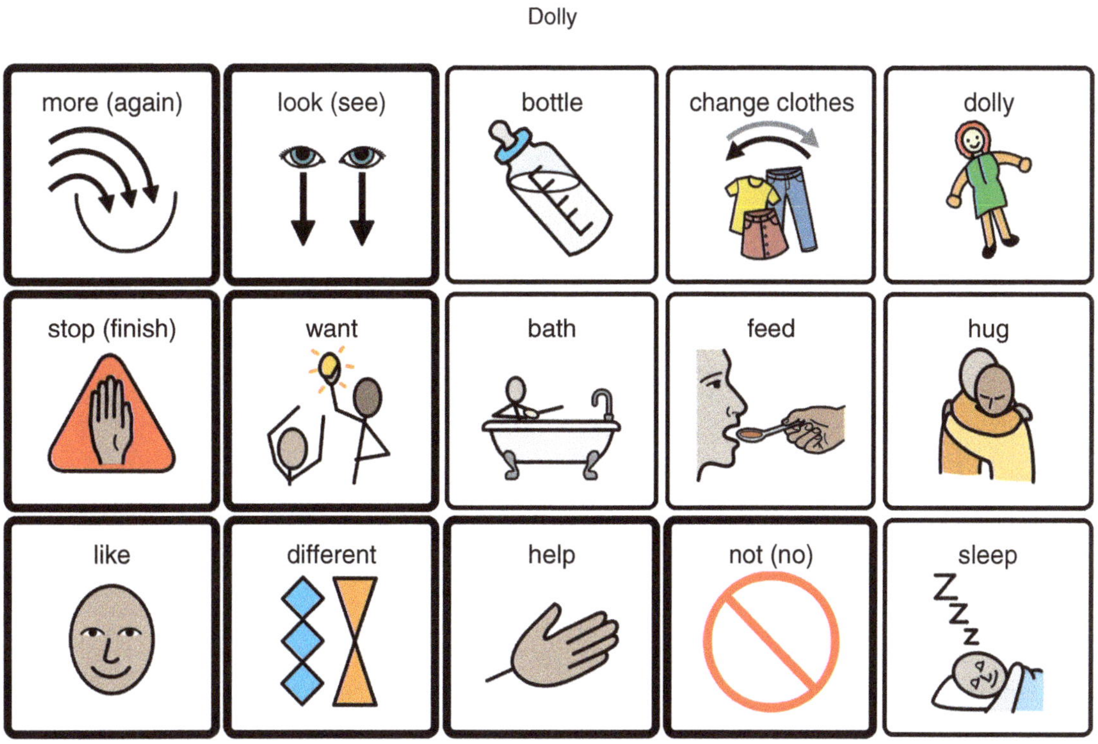

Figure 2.3 A dolly symbol chart.

Source: Created by the Ace Centre.

Communication Boards (Figure 2.3) and charts are often an individual page of symbols to support communication, consisting of both core and topic vocabulary. These often correspond to a given activity, for example, playing with dolls.

This image shows an example from Ace Centre.

Communication Books (Figure 2.4) provide bespoke pages of symbols, arranged in topics, to support a learner to communicate in different ways. These books can vary greatly in how they are organised – for example by size or number of symbols, as well as how they are accessed, for example, eye pointing, fist pointing, and so forth.

This image shows a range of paper-based PODD communication books.

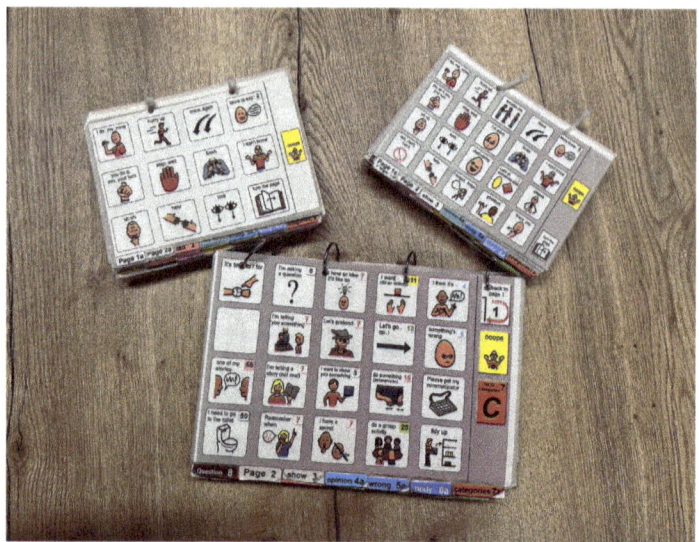

Figure 2.4 An image of three symbol books on a wooden surface.

Source: Photographed by the author.

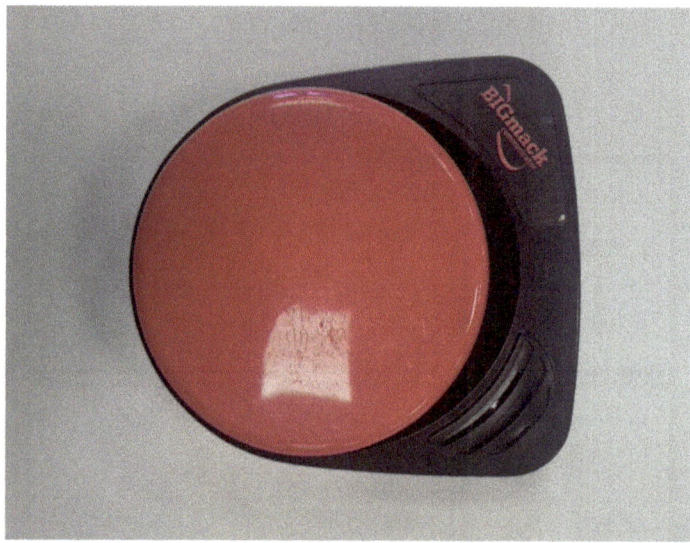

Figure 2.5 An image of single message VOCA with a red button on a black base.

Source: Photographed by the author.

Electronic AAC: Technology is also used to support AAC; these are often referred to as speech generating devices or voice output communication aids (VOCAs). Some examples of these include:

Single message devices (Figure 2.5) that enable the recording of a single message, which can then be played back when pressed.

Multiple message devices (Figure 2.6), which allow multiple words and messages to be stored.

This image shows an example of a GoTalk.

Electronic communication aids (Figure 2.7) with a dynamic nature can create complex and multiple messages. As with a communication book, these can vary greatly in how they are organised: for example by size or by the number of symbols, as well as by how these are accessed, for example, using a switch, joystick or eye gaze camera. (These alternative access methods will be discussed later in the book.)

This image shows an example of Proloquo2Go on an iPad.

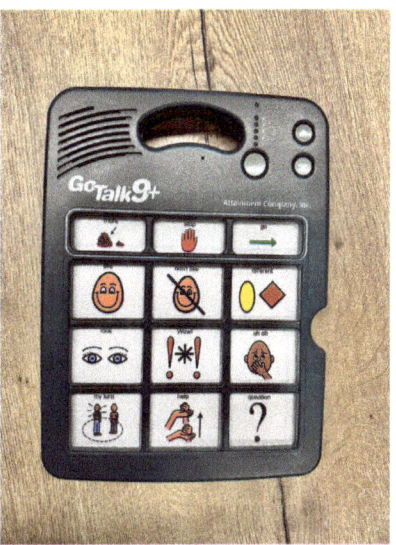

Figure 2.6 An image of a green device with 12 symbol pictures on it.

Source: Photographed by the author.

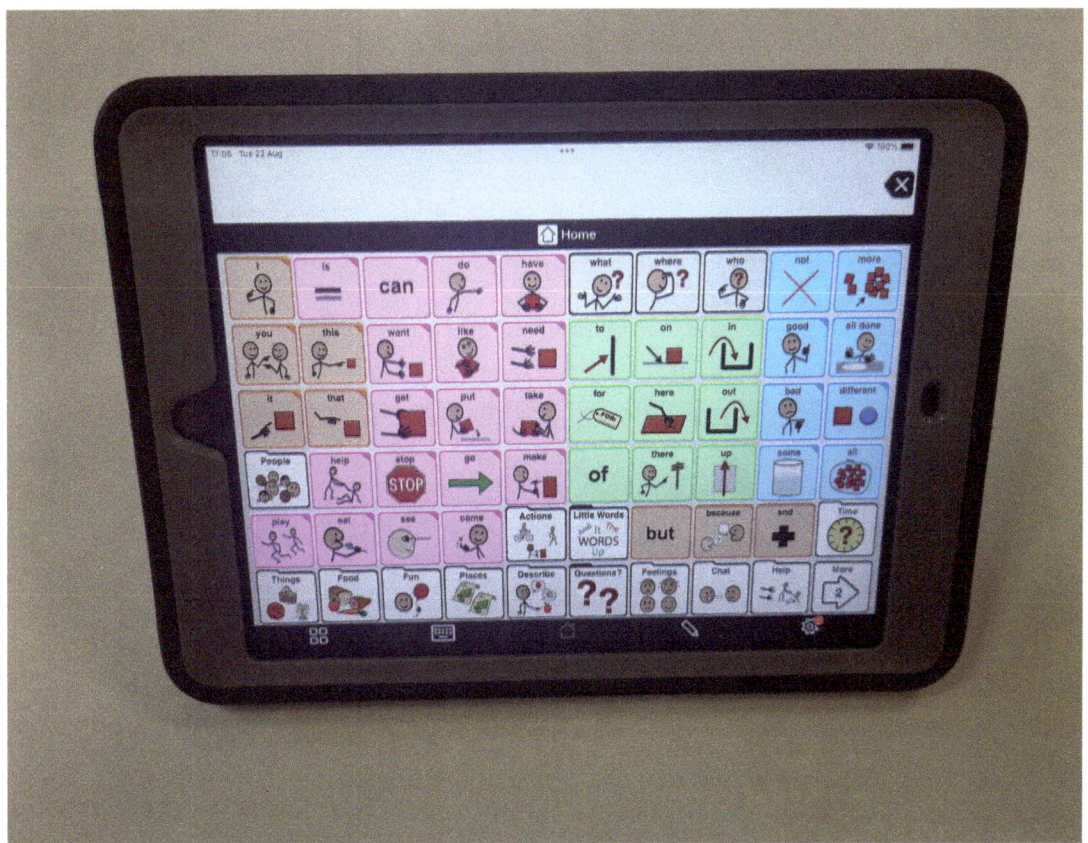

Figure 2.7 Image of an iPad with a visual display of a grid of symbols.

Source: Photographed by the author.

Specific Terminology used to Describe Features in Electronic AAC Systems and Communication Books

A symbol set is classified as the images used to represent given words. There are specific symbol sets produced by different AAC suppliers which are commercially available. Here are examples of how 'want' is represented from a selection of those symbol sets.

Figure 2.8 show examples of the Picture Communication Symbols (PCS), Widgit and SymbolStix symbol sets, which are the most commonly used symbol sets on both paper-based and electronic AAC.

A Page Set is classed as a group of communication pages. These can be organised into categories (categorized), according to the context (contextual), or according to the language (linguistically). This enables the learner to have efficient access to a broad vocabulary.

A vocabulary refers to the language available to the learner within the communication aid. We would always advocate for a robust vocabulary system, allowing learners an optimum chance of language development.

Figures 2.9–2.11 are examples of Proloquo2Go, SuperCore and TD Snap Core First on electronic AAC. These are all apps which can be downloaded onto an iPad.

The way these operate may be static, dynamic or a hybrid.

- *A Static Display* describes how the symbols are placed in a fixed location.
- *A Dynamic Display* describes the feature seen on some high-tech communication aids where pressing one cell will automatically open up another page.
- *A Hybrid Display* describes when there is a mixture of both these approaches.

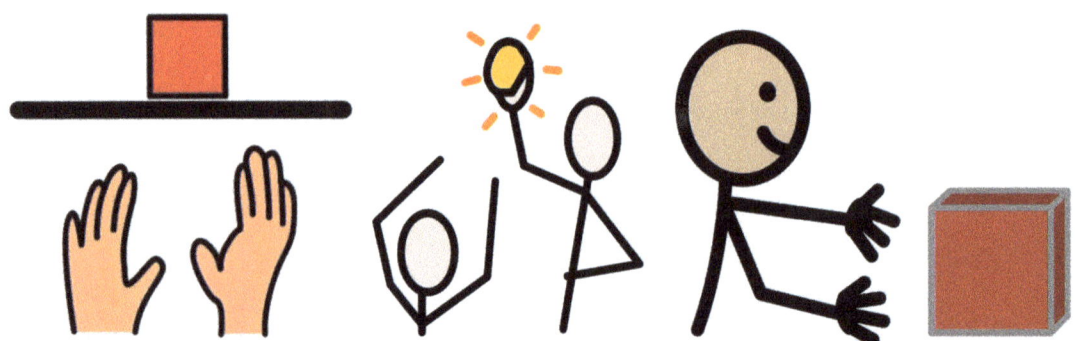

Figure 2.8 An image of three symbols.

Source: PCS and Boardmaker are trademarks of Tobii Dynavox LLC. All rights reserved. Used with permission. Widgit Symbols © Widgit Software Ltd 2002-2023 www.widgit.com. Used with permission. SymbolStix ® Copyright © 2023 SymbolStix, LLC. All rights reserved. Used with Permission.

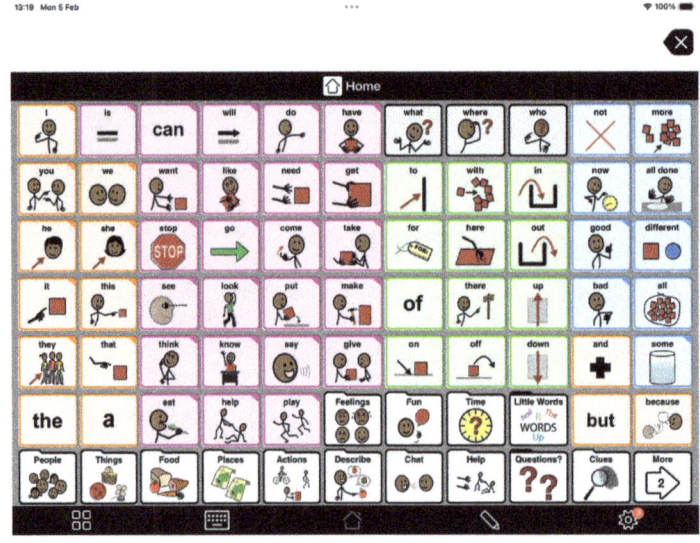

Figure 2.9 Screenshot of a grid of symbols with a black border on the top and bottom.

Source: www.assistiveware.com ©2019 AssistiveWare BV. All rights reserved. Symbols © 2019 SymbolStix, LLC.

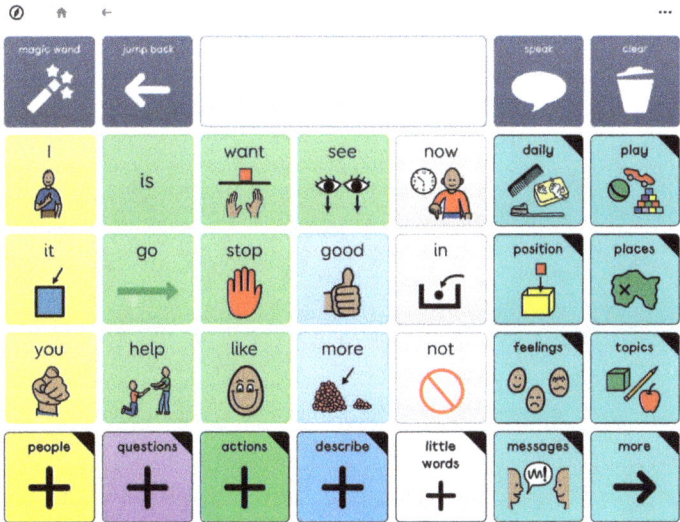

Figure 2.10 Screenshot of grid of symbols with a yellow column at the start.

Source: SmartBox, creators of Grid AAC software.

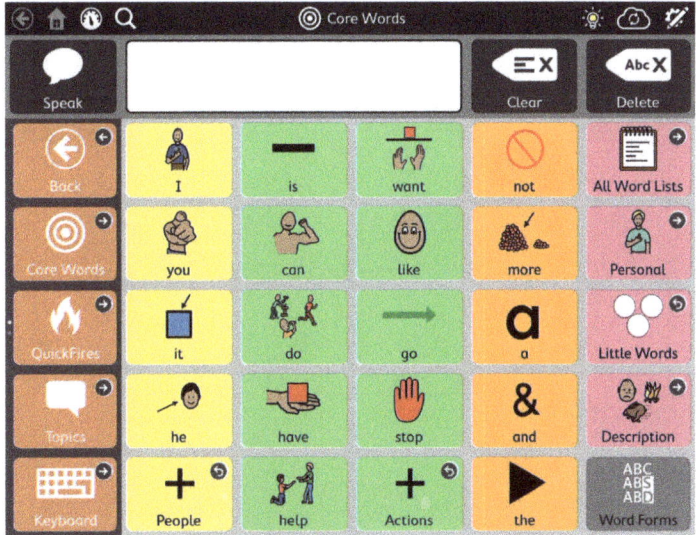

Figure 2.11 Screenshot of grid of symbols with and orange column at the start, taken from vocabulary. TD Snap, Core First vocabulary package.

Source: PCS and Boardmaker are trademarks of Tobii Dynavox LLC. All rights reserved. Used with permission.

Visual Scenes as shown in Figure 2.12 describes an approach where a photo or video represent a place, person or event, with corresponding vocabulary (usually phrases) available.

This example is from the WordPower vocabulary through Touch Chat, which is a communication app that can be downloaded onto an iPad.

Core and Fringe Vocabulary

Core vocabulary refers to a group of words which makes roughly 80 per cent of our communications. These are able to be used irrespective of the contexts. This includes words such as want, like, more, stop and help. These include a range of word types, for example pronouns, prepositions, adjectives and verbs, but very few nouns. You are unable to create a sentence without the use of core words. You can however create a sentence using only core words. These words often are hard to assign a symbol to as they are not pictographic. The symbols used can therefore seem very abstract. Many AAC systems have chosen to not symbolise core words. Due to this, these words need to be individually taught.

16 *Lifting the Veil of Terminology*

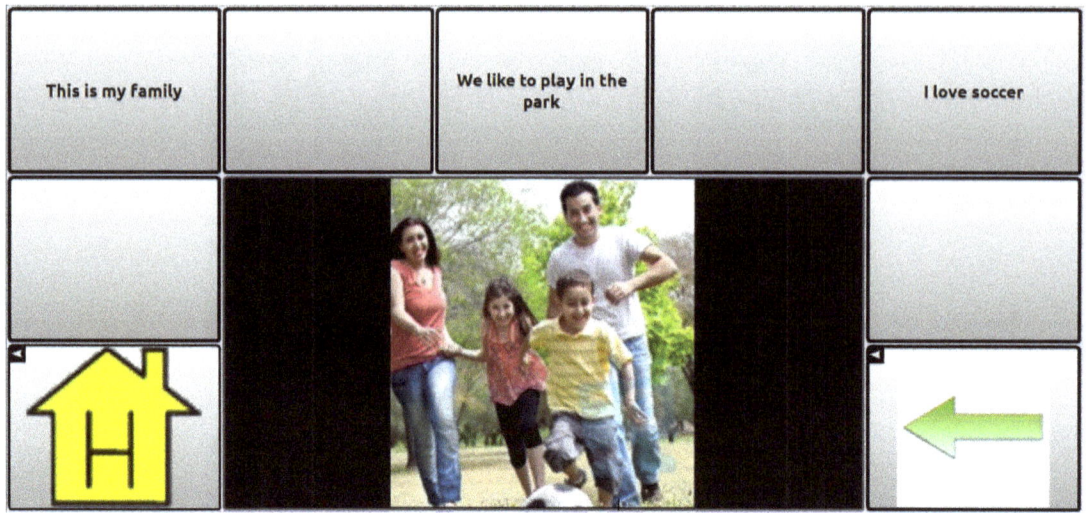

Figure 2.12 Screenshot of a picture of a family.

Source: Image from Liberator, Screenshot taken from vocabulary.

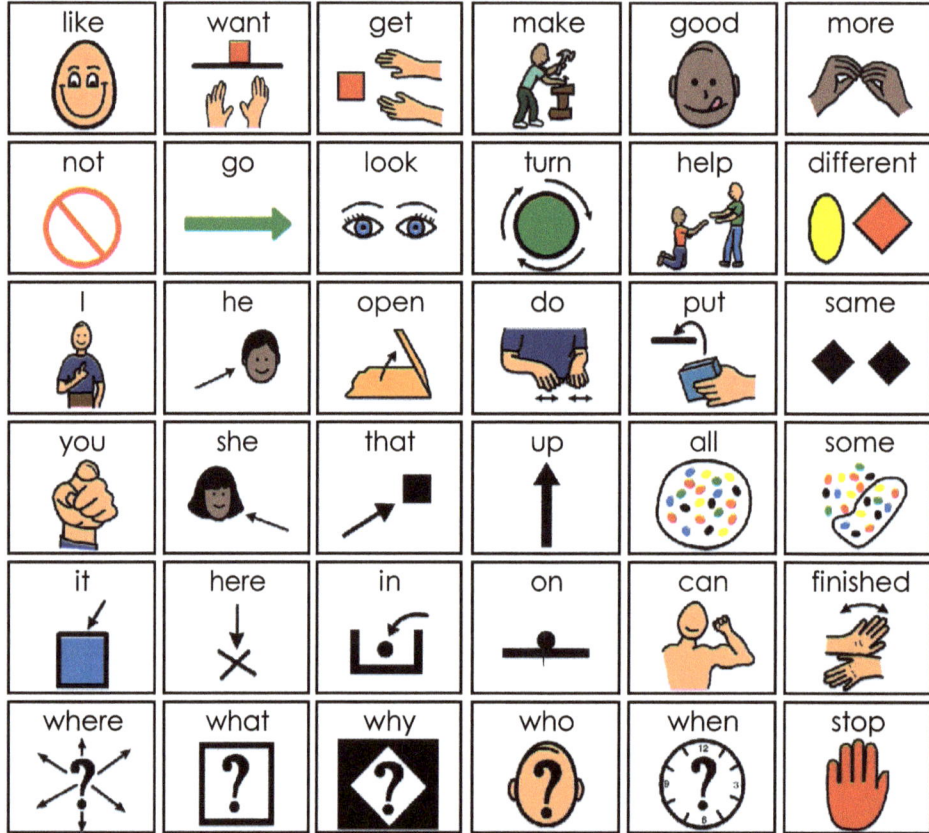

Figure 2.13 Image of 36 symbols on a white background.

Source: University of North Carolina at Chapel Hill, The Center for Literacy and Disability Studies, www.project-core.com.

Figure 2.13 is an example of a Project Core resource (an implementation model used to help educators support learners to access core vocabulary).

Discussion Point!

Imagine that you are going out shopping with friends. Using the Project Core 36 location board, how many different phrases could you say using this board? For example, 'want, go, here', 'like it', 'I like that', and so forth.

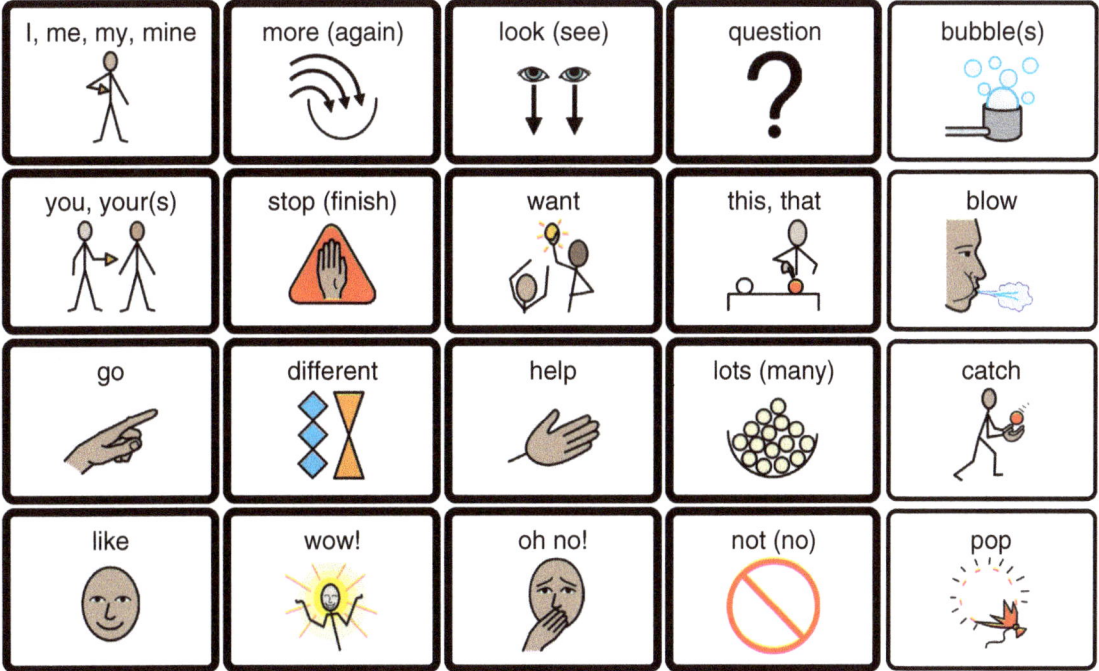

Figure 2.14 Image of 20 symbols with the title Bubbles.

Source: Created by the Ace centre https://acecentre.org.uk/resources

Fringe vocabulary refers to vocabulary that is specific to a given topic, environment, or learner. This cannot be used across contexts as seen with core vocabulary but can be combined with core vocabulary to create messages. Fringe words make up around 20 per cent of our daily spoken vocabulary but provides the rich detail which we are keen to share, as this is often around our interests and reflects what is important to us as individuals. There is huge variety in fringe vocabulary. Fringe words usually include nouns and proper nouns, including places, things and people. You are unable to create sentences using solely fringe vocabulary. As these words are more pictographic in nature, it is a lot simpler to assign a symbol to these, for example a symbol of a dog is easily recognisable as a dog.

Communication includes a mixture of both core and fringe vocabularies, both for learners who have verbal speech, as well as learners requiring aided language to support their expressive language, for example using AAC. By combining core and fringe vocabulary, the learner is also building their understanding of grammar and sentence structure.

Effective AAC systems should give access to both core and fringe vocabulary. There should be a focus on using these in combination, rather than just single words. The use of fringe vocabulary enables the construction of a more robust system for the learner. It is important to keep core vocabulary in a consistent location on each page within the AAC system.

Figure 2.14 is a simple resource created by Ace Centre to communicate during a bubbles activity, including both core vocabulary (e.g. more and stop) and fringe vocabulary (e.g. bubbles and blow).

Communication Partners

In addition to identifying terminology specific to AAC, it is also important to reflect on terms relating to the teaching and implementation of AAC.

Communication partners: These are any individuals who communicate and interact with the learner. This can include family, friends, educators and members of the community.

Figure 2.15 illustrates how lifelong communication partners, close friends and relatives are the closest and most common communication partners for a learner. You will often see learners using different communication methods based on where their communication partner fits within this image. For example, those close to the learner may be able to interpret the learner's speech,

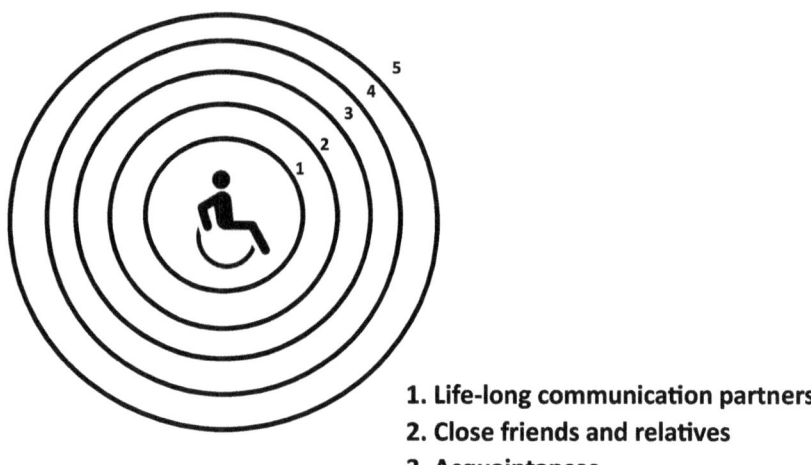

1. Life-long communication partners
2. Close friends and relatives
3. Acquaintances
4. Paid workers
5. Unfamiliar communication partners

Figure 2.15 Image of person in a wheelchair surrounded by five circles.

Source: Adapted from Blackstone's circle of communication partners (1999).

but unfamiliar partners find it far more challenging, so learners need to use AAC to get their message across with these unfamiliar communication partners.

Embedding good communication partner skills enable the learner to flourish. Simply giving the learner processing time enables time for the learner to absorb language and formulate a response.

Conclusion

This chapter has offered an overview to ensure you are equipped with some underpinning knowledge of specific terminology before continuing to read the rest of the book. As you work through the chapters, the terminology touched on in this chapter will be described in greater depth. It is important that terminology should never be a barrier, so having a shared language which is understood by all parties supporting the learner is a great place to start.

Introducing aided language/AAC into the classroom environment for learners with Speech, Language and Communication Needs can seem scary and overwhelming. In the next chapter the myths and misconceptions around the introduction of aided language/AAC will be explored. Having a deeper understanding of these will support you in facilitating discussions with other communication partners who may be reluctant, or too nervous, to introduce to aided language/AAC.

Bibliography

Department for Education and Department of Health (2015). *Special educational needs and disability code of practice: 0 to 25 years*. Available at: www.gov.uk/government/publications/send-code-of-practice-0-to-25 (Accessed: 14 January 2024)

International Society for Augmentive and Alternative Communication (2011). *What is AAC?* Available at: https://isaac-online.org/english/about-aac/ (Accessed: 14 January 2024)

Royal College of Speech and Language Therapists (2009). *What are speech, language and communication needs?*. Available at: www.rcslt.org/wp-content/uploads/media/Project/RCSLT/rcslt-communication-needs-factsheet.pdf (Accessed: 14 January 2024)

3 Myths and Misconceptions: What the Research Tells Us

You as a practitioner may face barriers from other educators or senior leaders within your organisation when introducing aided language into the classroom environment. That is why it's important for you to have the necessary information to validate your decision, especially if you find yourself in the position of doing this without access to the support and guidance of a speech and language therapist. Be reassured that research into the impact of the introduction of aided language shows that it will not hinder the development of natural speech.

> **Discussion Point!**
>
> - What barriers have you faced from other educators when you have tried to introduce aided language/AAC into your classroom practice?
> - If you can, take a moment to record the barriers you have faced. Then, at the end of the chapter, review which barriers could be negated by using the research shared to strengthen your reasoning for introducing aided language/AAC.

Questions may come from staff who are well established within the school or have worked with a particular learner with speech, language and communication needs for a significant amount of time, such as the learner's one-to-one support. Staff who typically challenge the use of aided language in the classroom often feel that they can understand the learner's expressive communication. These staff members feel that it is the responsibility of people around the learner with speech, language and communication needs to get to know them better. Familiar staff have tuned into any dysarthric (unclear) natural speech, or they know the learner so well that they can effectively interpret the learner's behaviours, gestures, and facial expressions. They therefore feel they can effectively advocate for the learner without the introduction of aided language. In this situation, it is positive that the learner has someone who can understand some, if not all, of their expressive communication. But it generally falls short when the staff team changes at points of transition, or when the learner has to communicate with less familiar communication partners. This can be a scary prospect for the learner, as suddenly they will experience an increase of communication breakdowns. This could be likened to moving to a new country every September and having to muddle through using a new language each year.

There are ways to prevent this situation, such as profiling and effectively documenting the expressive communication a learner uses. This can be done with the effective use of tools such as communication passports. When justifying the introduction of aided language, we need to be asking resistant staff members whether that learner can express everything that is in their head to anyone they want to share it with? That is autonomous communication. If the answer is no, then we need to give them access to aided language to facilitate this.

Romski and Sevcik (2005) produced an article highlighting some of the myths and misconceptions which may hinder the introduction of aided language/alternative, augmentative communication (AAC). You may be challenged with some of these myths and misconceptions when introducing aided language into the classroom.

Here are six myths that were addressed in the article:

Myth 1 AAC is a "last resort" in speech-language intervention.
Myth 2 AAC hinders or stops further speech development.
Myth 3 Children must have a certain set of skills to be able to benefit from AAC.
Myth 4 Speech-generating AAC devices are only for children with intact cognition.

Myth 5   Children have to be a certain age to be able to benefit from AAC.
Myth 6   There is a representational hierarchy of symbols from objects to written words (traditional orthography).

Myth 1: A 'Last Resort'

Aided language/alternative, augmentative communication (AAC) was identified as a tool to use once established that the learner's natural speech was unviable. It has now been identified that aided language/AAC can play an important role in minimising the risk of the learner experiencing communication failure. It is more important that the child can use expressive language effectively, rather than the emphasis being solely on speech production.

When thinking about introducing aided language/AAC into the classroom, educators and therapists alike can often hit an initial barrier. There can often be parental concern that the introduction of aided language/AAC will somehow hinder or stop the development of natural speech. When parents and carers hold this misconception, it can often lead to difficult conversations with families who perceive the introduction of aided language/AAC as a 'last resort'. This can leave parents and carers feeling as though everyone has given up hope that their child's verbal speech will develop. These are often the same families who have had many conversations with medical practitioners and have been told on numerous occasions what milestones their child has missed. Therefore, as a practitioner it is important to share with families what aided language/AAC will be introduced to support the learner's expressive communication and share the learner's successes.

We must lift the veil of the terminology of AAC and show families that aided language is not a massive step away from verbal communication. Rather, aided language/AAC is another aid to facilitate expressive communication. As educators, we know that we should do our utmost to support our learners to achieve their full potential, and we need to use every tool available to achieve this. So, when talking to families and carers about the introduction of aided language/AAC in the classroom to support a learner's expressive communication, we must be clear that aided language is another tool in the learner's toolkit to aid effective communication. The goal is to allow the learner to express whatever is in their head to anyone they want to share that with, and at any time. If we fall into the danger zone of waiting for natural speech to develop, whether that is the clarity of speech or speech production in general, and do not provide tools for learners to express themselves, there can be a significant impact on the mental health of that learner. They will often revert to using a suite of behaviours to communicate with those around them, some of which may be challenging and difficult to break once established.

Myth 2: A Hindrance to Natural Speech

For those learners who have some natural speech, it can often feel like introducing aided language/AAC could compromise the development of natural speech. Many practitioners follow a medical approach of 'use it or lose it', which often refers to a deterioration in muscles and skills when not used. Therefore, it can often feel like a dangerous road when aided language/AAC is introduced. Nobody wants to derail the verbal skills the learner has already achieved, so it's useful to read some of the research around this topic for reassurance.

One of the most cited research papers in how the use of AAC does not have a negative impact on the development of natural speech, is a research review carried out by Millar, Light and Schlosser (2006), which reviewed literature published between 1975 and 2003.

The review identified six studies which had enough methodological rigor for the best evidence analysis. These studies included children and adults with learning difficulties. The studies focused on interventions that involved instruction in manual signs or nonelectronic aided systems. The results from the research review found that 'None of the 27 cases demonstrated decreases in speech production as a result of AAC intervention, 11% showed no change, and the majority (89%) demonstrated gains in speech.'

Further research looked more specifically around AAC that was speech-generating and the positive impact that speech-generating AAC can have on the production of natural speech.

Support of Natural speech

Aspects of SGD use that may promote naural speech production

Communication effects	Motor effects	Acoustic effects
• Increase number of messages/functions • Increase number of conversational terms • Increase in utterance length	• Reduction in pressure to speak • Reduced physical demands	• Support for development of internal phonology • More natural to communication partner • Pairing of spokem with graphic symbols • Immediate output • Consistent across activation • Communcation across distance • Increase in number of speech models

Figure 3.1 Image of a 3-column table.

Source: Adapted from Blischak, Lombardino and Dyson, 'Use of Speech-Generating Devices: In Support of Natural Speech' (2003).

Sevcik et al. (1995) reported the results of a two-year research project that investigated the System for Augmented Language (SAL). In this project the participants used voice output communication aids (VOCAs). The results showed that seven of the thirteen project participants, including the 2 with autism, increased the proportion of spoken words in their vocabularies that were rated intelligible over the course of the project. The project raised questions around the impact that VOCAs contributed to the participants' verbal speech development. The researchers speculated that the consistent models of spoken words provided by the VOCAs immediately following each symbol selection may have had a positive impact.

Figure 3.1 highlights the effects of using a speech-generating device.

Looking at the positive acoustic effects of speech-generating devices highlighted by Blischak, Lombardino and Dyson – in the paper-based *Use of Speech-Generating Devices: In Support of Natural Speech* (2003) – we could take this further and also draw conclusions that using aided language which is presented in a paper-based format is equally as supportive, as the communication partner will often provide the speech model when making selections with the aided language/AAC system. The communication partner would become the tool to generate the speech model, rather than a device.

Myth 3: Children must have a certain Set of Skills to Benefit from AAC; Nobody is too Anything!

Another misconception that educators may face when introducing aided language into the classroom environment could be that the learner is not ready, or there are prerequisite skills that need to be completed before introducing aided language.

This links back to Piaget's stages of cognitive development (1936).

Stage	Age range	Presentation
Sensorimotor	0-2	Coordination of senses with motor responses and child will show sensory curiosity about the world. The language they will use is for demands and cataloguing. Object permanence is developed.
Preoperational	2-7	Symbolic thinking develops, along with the use of proper syntax and grammar to express concepts.
Concrete Operational	7-11	Concepts attached to concrete situations. Time, space and quantity are understood and can be applied, but not as independent concepts.
Formal Operational	11 years and older	Theoretical, hypothetical and counterfactual thinking. Abstract logic and reasoning are developed, strategy and planning are now able to be applied. Learned concepts can be applied in different contexts.

The focus here is on the latter developments in the Sensorimotor Stage and into the Preoperational Stage, where symbolic thinking develops. Learners who are classified as having profound and multiple learning difficulties are typically classified as working at the cognitive level of up to a two-year-old, which would link with the Sensorimotor Stage of cognitive development. Therefore, learners classed as having profound and multiple learning difficulties (PMLD) are perceived as unlikely to have the cognition required to have symbolic thinking, such as understanding that a photo of a cup represents a drink.

In reality, the classification of a PMLD learner is, in special school settings, often used to group learners who have physical and/or sensory disabilities and who are also nonverbal. As you can imagine this is a real danger zone to place a barrier around access to aided language based on an assumption of lack of cognition because the learner does not have the means to show what they know. Therefore, it is always best to take the stance of least dangerous assumption. Evidence has shown that educators can do no harm by introducing aided language/AAC to support expressive communication, at worse it has shown that it will have no impact, but at best we can help a learner to communicate.

The learner will also be older than two because they will be of school age. Due to this they will have experienced considerably more stimuli than that of a two-year-old, which could lead to a spikey profile of skills due to their physical/sensory disabilities. It is likely then that they will have cognition above that of a child at the Sensorimotor Stage of cognitive development.

Romski and Sevcik (2005) stated,

> there is also some evidence that severe physical disabilities and limited communication skills may interfere with the course of early cognitive development, in particular the development of object permanence and means-ends skills. Thus, developing language skills through AAC may be of critical importance if the individual is to make functional cognitive gains as well.
> (p. 180)

So rather than withholding access to aided language/AAC for that cohort of learners with the label PMLD need aided language input to support expressive communication more than many other groups of learners to also facilitate further cognitive development.

Myth 4: Speech-generating AAC Devices are only for Children with Intact Cognition

Some practitioners may hold historic views that learners who have more severe learning difficulties are less likely to be formulating large quantities of language in their heads. Due to this, the aided language the learner would require would be limited. Therefore, introducing a robust vocabulary package of aided language on a high-cost, speech-generating, electronic communication aid would not be cost effective.

However, AAC systems should always focus on the needs of each learner. Some learners do benefit from having a speech-generating device to hear the words being selected. There should be no cost restrictions on a learner accessing the aid that will best support their expressive communication. As we have moved into more recent times, technology is more readily available. As more mainstream technology, such as iPads are used as communication aids, electronic AAC is more affordable than ever before. This allows greater freedom for practitioners to choose the most appropriate communication system to support the learner's expressive communication, whether that is a printed communication book or a speech-generating device.

Myth 5: Children have to be a certain Age to be able to Benefit from AAC

Parents often take infants to baby signing classes. These are promoted as a fun way for you to learn some sign language with your baby so you can communicate together before they can talk. No parent or carer entering those classes thinks that their child will never speak if they start signing to each other. Rather, they are keen to communicate with their child from an early age and want their child to express themselves in a manner which can be clearly understood. The introduction of aided language/AAC should be perceived the same way. Communication partners want to know what children are thinking, and this is a tool for them to share the language they are generating in their heads.

When we look at typical language development, we can see that the communicative functions of language develop at an early age (Figure 3.2). If a learner does not have the verbal language to match typical communication development, then aided language/AAC needs to be introduced to give them access to a language they can use to support expressive communication. We are not expecting the child to be a fluent user of language at an early age. However, they do need access to a language they can use if verbal language isn't a viable option for them to fully express themselves. Therefore, we need to give the learner access to aided language/AAC, so language functions continue to develop. Language development should not be hindered due to the lack of access to a mode of communication.

Myth 6: There is a Representational Hierarchy of Symbols from Objects to Written Words (Traditional Orthography)

For many years the representational hierarchy has been practiced in schools (Figure 3.3). There was a shared understanding that a learner needed to begin at the first stage of the hierarchy, using real objects to represent something before they could progress onto using photographs, symbols and then written words to support expressive communication.

Using a child's own cup to ask them if they want a drink is meaningful to them and a child will make the connection between their cup and them getting a drink quickly, as parents and carers will constantly reinforce the connection between the drink and the cup throughout the day. Likewise, a photograph of mum is easily identifiable as mum, as the child sees mum's image frequently, and everyone is always attributing meaning to that image by saying 'is that mum/mummy?'

This is why many educators will feel like there is a need for personalised photographs when introducing aided language/AAC in the classroom. Personalisation is extremely powerful for a learner, as there is already a lot of prior in-context learning that has occurred to understand that their cup means drink, or the photograph represents mummy. This activity has been repeated time and time again every day.

Limitations of using objects or photographs begin when they are used to represent in a more general way. How could a learner talk about their friend's mum when all they have access to is a photograph of their own mum?

Gayle Porter and Linda Burkhart, in their article, 'Limitations with Using a Representational Hierarchy Approach for Language Learning' (2010), highlight that 'more concrete representations such as objects and photos can actually make the use of these as symbols for communication purposes more difficult. E.g., [a]s the photo of a particular cup visually has so much in common with just that cup[,] it can be very difficult to use it to represent the more general concept of drink (which may come in any number of cups).'

Objects and photographs typically represent nouns and, by their very nature, can often lead educators to offer access to nouns only for expressive communication. By doing this it is easy to fall into the trap that choice making is all we can offer that learner, which then becomes a choice board. On top of this, think of all the possible things they may want to choose in any given context and imagine getting a personalised photo or object for each one. The task soon becomes overwhelming and impossible to facilitate. Who carries around all of those objects with the learner all day long? The reality is, the number of objects of reference offered is generally small and therefore significantly limiting the aided language being offered to the learner.

We know that language develops best in learning to communicate and learning language in natural contexts, then thinking about what that typical communication development looks like.

When we look at how a child develops language, we can see that some of the earliest communication functions are things that cannot easily be represented by objects or photographs, such as rejecting, protesting and seeking attention. These can be represented, although in an abstract manner, using graphic symbols (Figure 3.4).

Graphic symbols are often perceived as too complex for some learners, particularly a learner who is younger or diagnosed as having a learning disability. However, we cannot give learners

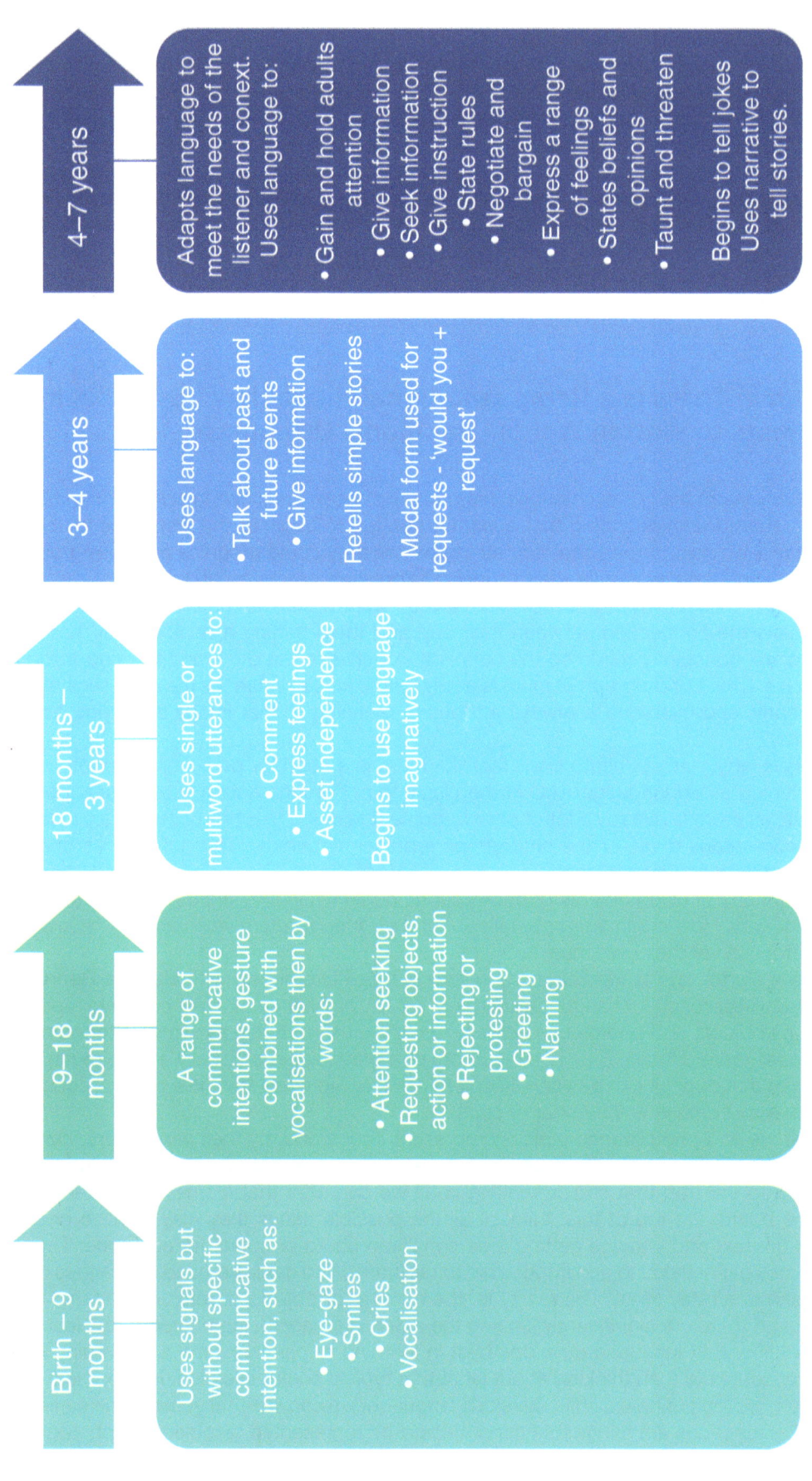

Figure 3.2 An image of 5 developmental stages.
Source: Created by the author.

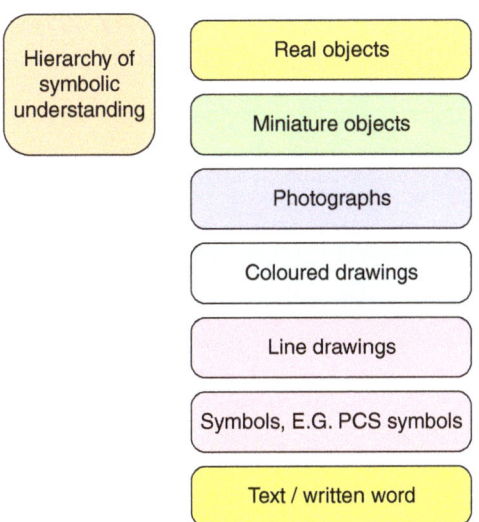

Figure 3.3 An image showing 7 stages in a column format.

Source: Created by the author.

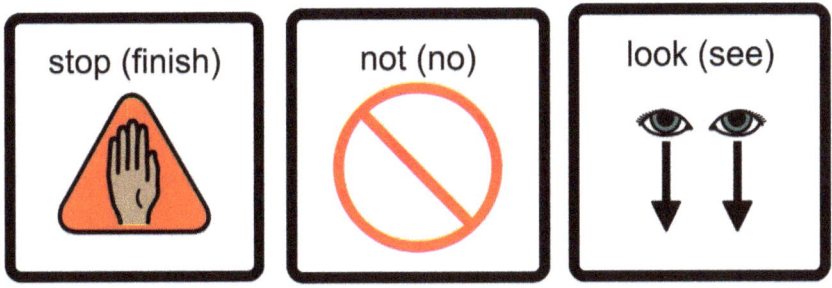

Figure 3.4 An image of 3 symbols.

Source: PCS and Boardmaker are trademarks of Tobii Dynavox LLC. All rights reserved. Used with permission.

access to a symbol-based vocabulary and just expect them to guess the meaning. Some symbols by their very nature are easy to guess and make meaningful connections, as they are more iconic, for example, a symbol of a dog is easy to match to a dog. However, we know that the earliest communicative functions are not nouns that are easily represented. Therefore, to give our learners the same opportunities for language learning, we have to ensure that they are taught aided language that can represent those abstract language functions, too. These are generally classed as core vocabulary words and, at the earliest stages of language development, they include words such as no, mine, more, stop. We would also expect to see the learner use some of the noun-based fringe vocabulary for the language function of naming, for example, a learner saying 'dog' when pointing to a dog.

If we sit firmly in the structure of the representational hierarchy, there is a danger that learners will not be taught those earliest language functions, such as rejecting, as they are difficult to represent with objects of reference and photographs. This narrows communication to [CEchoice] making, which is not the same as a learner using autonomous communication. This is unlikely to stimulate language acquisition. "The aim is to stimulate communication and language development to support children in learning to communicate for the same purposes and functions as their speaking peers" (Gayle Porter and Linda Burkhart, 2010).

Conclusion

This chapter focussed on the article written by Romski and Sevcik (2005), which highlighted seven myths and misconceptions which may hinder the introduction of aided language/AAC. It explored key theories, such as: the 'Hierarchy of Symbolic Understanding'; Piaget's 'Stages of

Cognitive Development'; and the 'Pragmatic Profile of Early Communication Skills' (Dewart and Summers, 1995) – all of which have had impact on who we perceive aided language/AAC may be appropriate for.

The following chapter will discuss the importance of teamwork to introduce a learner to aided language/AAC.

Bibliography

Blischak, D., Lombardino, L. and Dyson, A. (2003). Use of Speech-Generating Devices: In Support of Natural Speech. *Augmentative and Alternative Communication*, 19(1), pp.29–35. doi: https://doi.org/10.1080/0743461032000056478

Dewart, H. and Summers, S. (1995). *The pragmatics profile of everyday communication skills in children*. Windsor: Nfer-Nelson.

Millar, D.C., Light, J.C. and Schlosser, R.W. (2006). The Impact of Augmentative and Alternative Communication Intervention on the Speech Production of Individuals With Developmental Disabilities: A Research Review. *Journal of Speech, Language, and Hearing Research*, 49(2), pp.248–264. doi: https://doi.org/10.1044/1092-4388(2006/021)

Piaget, J. (1936). *Origins of intelligence in the child*. London: Routledge & Kegan Paul.

Porter, G. and Burkhart, L. (2010). *Limitations with Using a Representational Hierarchy Approach for Language Learning*. Available at: https://lindaburkhart.com/wp-content/uploads/2016/07/representational_hierarchy_draft.pdf (Accessed: 22 April 2024).

Romski, M. and Sevcik, R.A. (2005). Augmentative Communication and Early Intervention. *Infants & Young Children*, 18(3), pp.174–185. doi: https://doi.org/10.1097/00001163-200507000-00002

scholar.google.co.uk. (n.d.). *Google Scholar*. [online] Available at: https://scholar.google.co.uk/scholar?q=Limitations+with+Using+a+Representational+Hierarchy+Approach+for+Language+Learning&hl=en&as_sdt=0&as_vis=1&oi=scholart (Accessed 14 Jan. 2024).

Sevcik, R.A., Romski, M.A., Watkins, R.V. and Deffebach, K.P. (1995). Adult Partner-Augmented Communication Input to Youth With Mental Retardation Using the System for Augmenting Language (SAL). *Journal of Speech, Language, and Hearing Research*, 38(4), pp.902–912. doi: https://doi.org/10.1044/jshr.3804.902

4 Education Is Not an Island: The Importance of Teamwork

Supporting learners with Speech, Language and Communication Needs (SLCN) within a classroom setting can often feel overwhelming, particularly for early-career teachers who have had limited instruction around teaching Special Educational Needs and Disabilities as part of their initial teacher training. Without educators having access to the underpinning knowledge, they are left feeling isolated and not knowing where to begin, despite having the best intentions. Learners with SLCN are so diverse that it can seem impossible to know what will work best for individuals and how to implement it. Drawing solely upon their classroom experience can cause education to be seen as an isolated island, rather than a community, rich in professionals who collaborate and engage in teamwork to meet the needs of learners.

Speech and language therapists play a fundamental role in supporting learners with SLCN, however, due to the national shortage of speech and language therapists there is often limited support, with referral waiting lists ever increasing, whilst trends are showing an increase in learners identified with a primary need of speech, language and communication needs (Speech and Language UK, 2023). Where speech and language therapists previously had the resources and capacity to work closely alongside pupils with speech, language and communication needs, in the current climate, input often can involve assessment and diagnosis, leading to target setting, for learners to then be discharged without any ongoing support being offered. This leads to pressure being placed upon teaching staff to meet the needs of learners with SLCN.

To best meet the needs of learners with SLCN, collaborative working is key. This can take many forms; some key examples are considered below.

Joint Assessment Process

Due to the current impact of Speech and Language Therapy provision, Speech and language therapists working in isolation to assess learners can have little impact on ongoing implementation within the classroom environment once their involvement has ceased. This can cause Speech and Language Therapy and Education to act as two distinct entities, rather than working in collaboration to improve outcomes for learners with SLCN. A national shortage of speech and language therapists has caused them to be stretched, with less capacity to work directly with learners. This can have considerable implications in terms of assessing learners identified as presenting with SLCN. There is an increased need to draw on professionals working closely with learners, including teaching and support staff, as well as parents, to gain a true profile of the learner. This collaborative working enables a holistic view of the learner, considering their presentation across environments.

This collaborative working can have a much further reaching impact than Speech and language therapists working separate from Education. This can enable all professionals working with the learner to be on the 'same page', enabling a realistic profile of the learner, leading to greater personalisation in goal setting.

Joint Target Setting

As a result of joint working to assess a learner with SLCN, personalised targets can be set jointly. This has a positive impact on the learner's outcomes, as these targets will consider the environments to which the learner is exposed, and how they present in these. Education staff have a detailed understanding of how the learner interacts in the classroom environment and will be able to identify realistic opportunities to practise skills within the school setting.

DOI: 10.4324/9781003410836-4

Likewise, educators target setting for a learner in isolation from speech and language therapists, can experience challenges in setting appropriate targets due to a lack of underpinning knowledge of speech and language therapy.

Interventions

Learners with SLCN may engage in 1:1 intervention, often administered by support staff, to focus on speech and language targets. However, there can often be limited opportunities to build on these skills, generalising them back into the classroom environment and their everyday life.

This lack of generalisation can make interventions not be valued and considered worthwhile for learners, being squeezed into the timetable, removing the learner from school life and causing them to not feel fully included within classroom activities. This is often particularly true in mainstream settings where there may be one or two learners in the classroom with SLCN.

Support staff who frequently implement interventions can often have less experience than teaching staff in supporting learners with Speech Language and Communication Needs. Unlike teachers who will have had some training on how to support learners with SLCN, support staff often enter the classroom without any prior experience. Therefore, it is key that all staff carrying out interventions with a learner are involved in the assessment and target setting process with speech and language therapists ensuring that support staff carrying out interventions gain a deeper understanding of elements being taught and the reasoning behind these.

Special Educational Needs Co-ordinators (SENCOs), particularly within mainstream settings, are often involved in interactions with speech and language therapists. This offers teachers support at a more managerial level and can ensure relevant support is in place for the learner, to enable targets to be worked on. This adds to the collaborative working within the school setting, with teachers and support staff feeling less alone as they have support from a staff member who most likely will have prior experience of supporting learners with Speech Language and Communication Needs.

Despite school staff and speech and language therapists working in collaboration and with joint meetings, this still does not tackle the issue of interventions taking place in isolation. To truly enable the optimal impact of targets, these should be integrated throughout the learner's day. The support of a speech and language therapist in working alongside classroom staff can be integral to its effectiveness. When all stakeholders work collaboratively to identify opportunities to work on goals, this can have a far greater impact than isolated sessions.

Peers are an incredibly powerful tool to use to support learners with SLCN. Peer modelling has been identified as having more significant impact than solely working with staff (Thiemann-Bourque, Feldmiller, Hoffman, and Johnera, 2018). This provides more natural interactions, again, enabling generalisation of skills. By working with peers, learning can more readily be taken outside of the classroom context – for example, when playing in the playground.

To further enable generalisation into everyday life for the learner, the parents and carers play a pivotal role in ensuring this extends outside the school environment to the home environment, in the community, interacting with family, friends and unfamiliar communication partners. If the targets are set in partnership with parents, carers and family members, their engagement, as well as the learners, will likely increase. By making the implementation more dynamic and linked to the child's interests and motivators, parents and carers are far more likely to work on targets at home rather than isolated activities without any context. Children spend only 30 hrs a week at school, so integration of interventions into the home environment can have a significant impact.

Figure 4.1 highlights how, if the delivery of an intervention is solely within a speech and language therapy session, it is likely to have less impact, because it is infrequent. However, if intervention is integrated into classroom practice and the home environment, this can have increased opportunities to practice skills and have greater impact.

Reviewing Targets

The initial joint target-setting with the speech and language therapist is often not continued on an on-going basis, causing the team around the child to lose their way in terms of next steps,

	Monday	Tuesday	Wednesday	Thursday	Friday	Saturday	Sunday
7 am	Home	Home	Home	Home	Home	Home	Home
8 am	Home	Home	Home	Home	Home	Home	Home
9 am	SaLT	School	School	School	School	Home	Home
10 am	School	School	School	School	School	Home	Home
11 am	School	School	School	School	School	Home	Home
12 pm	School	School	School	School	School	Home	Home
1 pm	School	School	School	School	School	Home	Home
2 pm	School	School	School	School	School	Home	Home
3 pm	School	School	School	School	School	Home	Home
4 pm	Home	Home	Home	Home	Home	Home	Home
5 pm	Home	Home	Home	Home	Home	Home	Home
6 pm	Home	Home	Home	Home	Home	Home	Home
7 pm	Home	Home	Home	Home	Home	Home	Home
8 pm	Home	Home	Home	Home	Home	Home	Home
9 pm	Home	Home	Home	Home	Home	Home	Home
10 pm	Home	Home	Home	Home	Home	Home	Home

Figure 4.1 A table splitting up the times of day.

Source: Created by the author.

as they do not have the specialist skills of a speech and language therapist. Due to this, regular collaborative reviews are necessary.

These meetings will enable targets to be reviewed, and next steps to be identified so the therapy does not lose momentum over time. In an ideal world speech and language therapists will have ongoing reviews with the learner and supporting team to review the learner's current skills and how to move forward – however, this is sadly not consistent nationally. Due to this, it is important school staff, parents and carers are confident in knowing the procedure to refer into speech and language therapy services, and when this may be appropriate. General Practitioners are the gatekeepers to making referrals back into health services, however this can also be initiated by school staff, for example SENCOs in some areas. This process can be notably more seamless if the learner is within a specialist setting, where Speech and language therapists are often available on site, in contrast to in mainstream settings, where Speech and language therapists often see learners within clinical hospital settings, rather than within the school environment.

Despite the involvement and collaboration of Speech and language therapists, school staff (including SENCOs, teachers and support staff) and parents and carers, in some circumstances this continues to look at one aspect of skill development in isolation, rather than a more holistic view of the learner.

Integrated Therapy Reviews

Some learners with Speech Language and Communication Needs have co-occurring difficulties, including physical disabilities. This can be particularly true for those with complex communication needs. These learners have the input of wider professionals than just speech and language therapists, for example physiotherapists (PT) and occupational therapists (OT). Due to this, many NHS trusts have moved away from separate reviews by speech and language therapists, PT and OTs, instead engaging in integrated therapy reviews. This working together ensures targets set consider the perspective of a range of professionals and how to holistically ensure the learner's needs are met and progress is made.

Education, Health and Care Plans

Most of the learners one comes across with SLCNs have their needs met via SEN Support within a mainstream school. Some, however, may require an Education, Health and Care Plan (EHCP), as identified in DfE SEND Code of Practice (2015) to be put in place and thus have additional support within their setting, or will be educated within a more specialist setting. As part of the process of gaining an EHCP, the views of a range of professionals are sought in order to enable a holistic picture of the learner. These can include:

- Educators
- Parents and carers
- Paediatricians
- Social workers
- Speech and language therapists, physiotherapists or occupational therapists
- Educational psychologists

Reviews of the Education Health Care Plans are held annually; however, it is incredibly rare for all those professionals working with the individual to attend these and input in a collaborative manner. Plans are reviewed, and changes can be requested following reviews, particularly at points of transition. However, plans can often be outdated and no longer reflect the needs and presentation of the learner (DfE, 2020). For the learner, this can often lead to complications at transition points.

> **Discussion Point!**
>
> - Your learners with Speech Language and Communication Needs may have many different professionals who are supporting them.
> - How do you share this information with communication partners who may be less familiar?

Communication Passports

One way to ensure information is shared effectively at transition points is the use of up-to-date communication passports. These are an invaluable tool to support learners with SLCN. This person-centred booklet pulls together information regarding the learner and presents the subject in a user-friendly format. These can be used across settings and play a key role in ensuring continuity in provision and care.

Sally Miller created a template of a communication passport in partnership with Call Scotland (2003), which can be accessed here: www.communicationpassports.org.uk/creating-passports/

Figures 4.2 and 4.3 are examples from the basic communication passport and adult communication passport:

These can take several different formats and be presented in a variety of user-friendly ways. A further example can be seen on the following page. As these are individual and unique to everyone, they can be easily adapted and tailored to suit the individual and the environment they are in. What works for one individual and their setting may not be as successful with a different individual or alternative setting.

The use of a communication passport gives the learner a vehicle to share information about themselves. Figures 4.4 and 4.5 written in the first person hence, giving the learner a voice to talk about themselves in a way that is easily understood by others. It is important to ensure the learner is an active participant when the passport is created, rather than being something created solely by professionals. Learners can play a role in choosing pictures and photos to show what is important to them. It is also helpful to include parents and carers in creating a communication passport.

Parents interact with a vast array of professionals to support their children. Communication passports are a great way to share information in a quick, easily digestible manner, making them perfect for busy appointments so parents and carers do not need to repeat themselves at each appointment. Should learners require for example a hospital stay or respite, these are far more effective to use than printing the whole EHCP for staff. Retaining information contained within an EHCP can be incredibly challenging due to the length of the document.

By ensuring that the communication passport is easily accessible, this can be used in the moment by staff working with the learner, both externally and within the school environment. This will ensure everyone working with the learner is using a consistent approach, which can reduce the frustration of a learner with a speech, language and communication need.

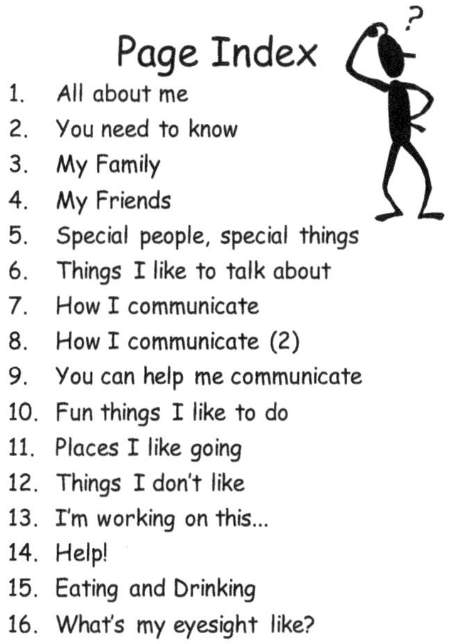

Page Index

1. All about me
2. You need to know
3. My Family
4. My Friends
5. Special people, special things
6. Things I like to talk about
7. How I communicate
8. How I communicate (2)
9. You can help me communicate
10. Fun things I like to do
11. Places I like going
12. Things I don't like
13. I'm working on this...
14. Help!
15. Eating and Drinking
16. What's my eyesight like?

Figure 4.2 An image showing a confused stick man with the title page index.

Source: Created by Call Scotland. www.callscotland.org.uk

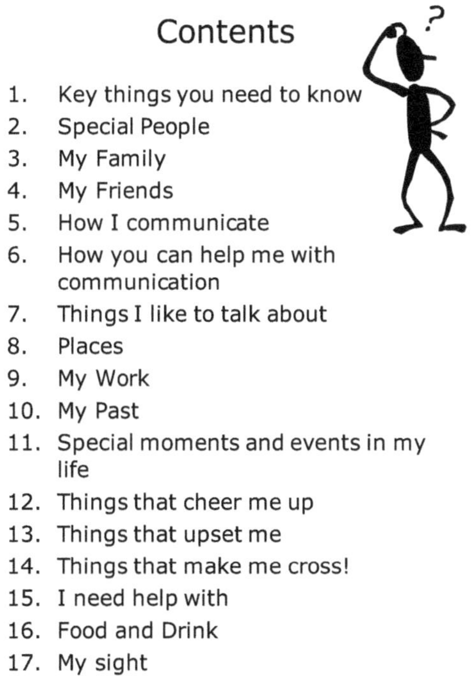

Contents

1. Key things you need to know
2. Special People
3. My Family
4. My Friends
5. How I communicate
6. How you can help me with communication
7. Things I like to talk about
8. Places
9. My Work
10. My Past
11. Special moments and events in my life
12. Things that cheer me up
13. Things that upset me
14. Things that make me cross!
15. I need help with
16. Food and Drink
17. My sight

Figure 4.3 An image showing a confused stick man with the title contents.

Source: Created by Call Scotland. www.callscotland.org.uk/

Benefits of Communication Passports

A communication passport can benefit both the learner and those working with them. Here are some of the benefits:

- It shares information of the learner's preferred communication methods and systems, which those working with the learner can quickly access.
- It can accompany the learner wherever they go, ensuring the team around the learner know important information about how to best support them.
- As the learner is actively involved in creating the passport and generating ideas, this ensures that it is truly bespoke to the learner and their likes and interests.

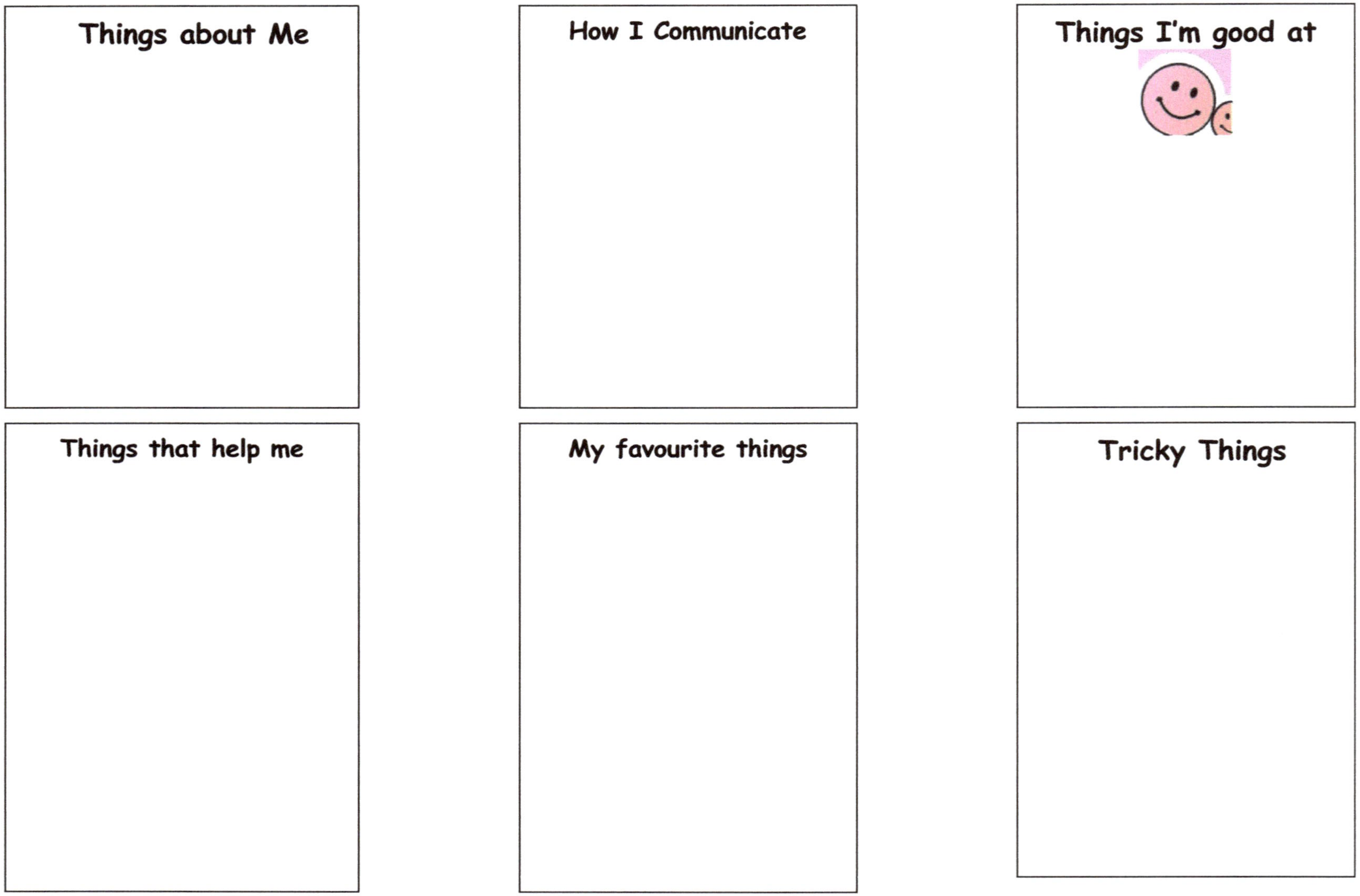

32 Education Is Not an Island: The Importance of Teamwork

Things I'm good at	Tricky Things

How I Communicate	My favourite things

Things about Me	Things that help me

Figure 4.4 This shows 6 boxes about a person with clipart images.

Source: Created by Call Scotland www.callscotland.org.uk/

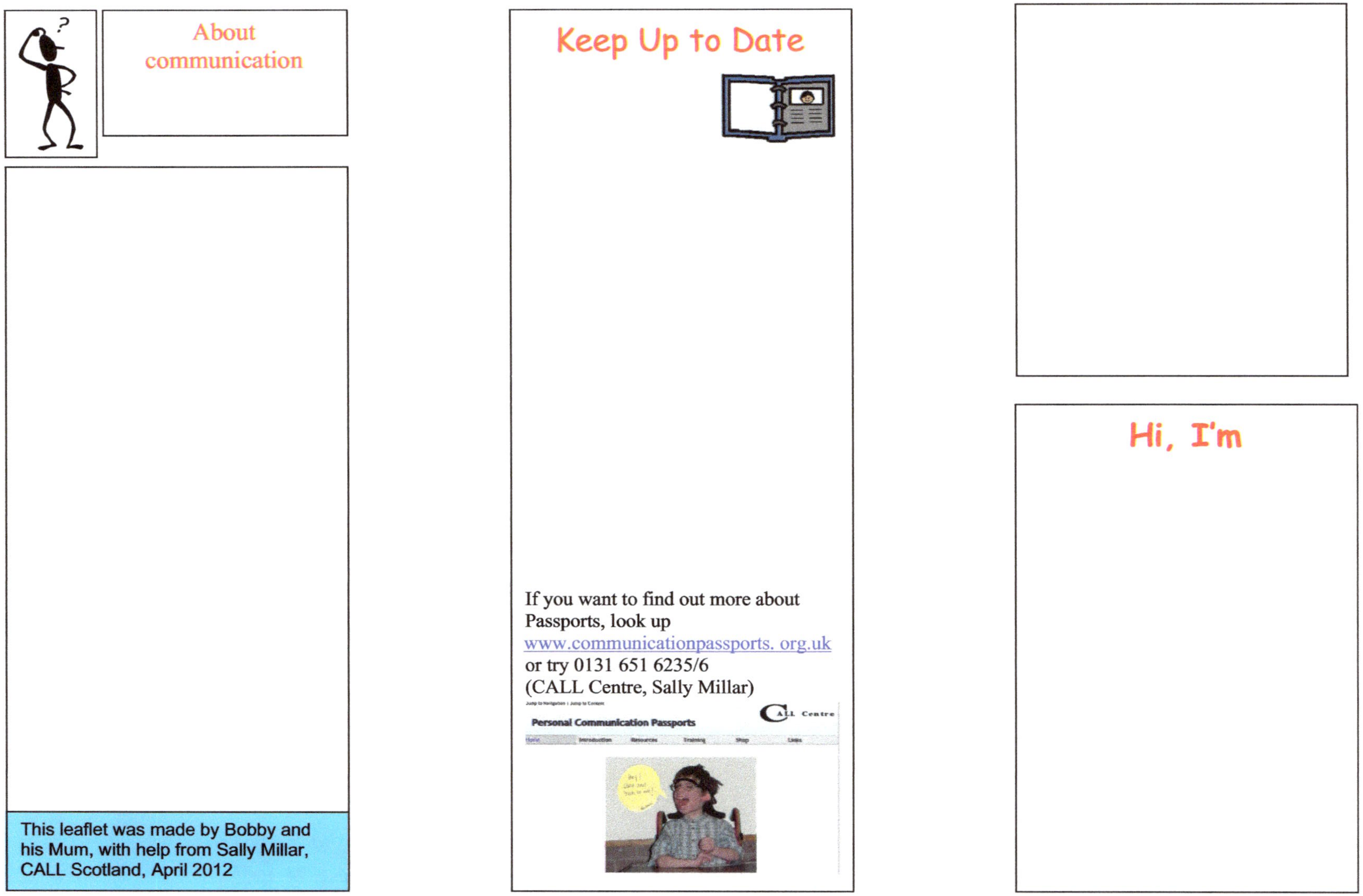

Education Is Not an Island: The Importance of Teamwork 33

Hi, I'm

Keep Up to Date

If you want to find out more about Passports, look up www.communicationpassports.org.uk or try 0131 651 6235/6 (CALL Centre, Sally Millar)

About communication

This leaflet was made by Bobby and his Mum, with help from Sally Millar, CALL Scotland, April 2012

Figure 4.5 This shows 3 boxes with a clipart picture of a person.
Source: Created by Call Scotland www.callscotland.org.uk/

- The passport is a working document, so over time this will evolve as the learner's needs may change and interests may vary. This updated information is easily accessible to the team around the learner if the simple structure of the passport is retained.
- This can lower the anxiety of the learner, as all those supporting can provide consistent support.
- The passport empowers staff to interact with the learner and respond in a manner that is helpful for the learner and enables them to reach their potential and actively engage. This can provide strategies to support the learner's receptive and expressive language and therefore enables the communication partners to adapt and change their interactions accordingly.
- It enhances inter-agency planning and collaboration, enabling improved consistency and continuity of support for the learner irrespective of the context they are faced with. This working together is integral in meeting the needs of the learner.
- Within the school environment, it enables unfamiliar staff, such as supply staff, new staff and volunteers to gain essential information for effective communication with the learner.
- The passport can identify any gaps in support and provision, which can feed back into the review process of any speech and language therapy targets set.

One of the instances in which communication passports can have the greatest impact is at times of transition. Communication passports provide professionals the opportunity to gain information about the needs of the learner prior to working with them. Without such a document the individual may not have access to their communication system to enable communication with those around them. When transitioning from one classroom to the next without information being shared, with key documents such as communication passports, support strategies may be missed, and learners can then appear to have regressed. The six-week summer holidays are often attributed to an individual appearing to lose skills, or this could be attributed to the new team not having the necessary information on how to best facilitate the learner's communication.

Discussions may happen informally between the individuals in different class teams; however, this information is not always retained and can often be subjective. Using a communication passport ensures that things are consistently followed through to enable a smooth transition.

On a larger scale this can support the learner's transition into different settings and ultimately into adulthood, as they work with a range of professionals and people. The stumbling point in transitions is often moving from child to adult services. This can be a huge jump for learners, with their care being moved from one service to another.

Conclusion

This chapter explored the importance of professionals working together as part of a multidisciplinary team to meet the needs of learners with Speech, Language and Communication Needs to engage in joint assessment and target setting. This chapter highlighted the importance of information sharing and gave examples on how you can facilitate this through resources such as communication passports.

Next we will consider some of the barriers you may face in real life implementation in the classroom. The next chapter will look at research into AAC abandonment and reflect on ways to avoid this.

Bibliography

Department for Education and Department of Health (2015). *Special educational needs and disability code of practice: 0 to 25 years*. Available at: www.gov.uk/government/publications/send-code-of-practice-0-to-25 (Accessed: 14 January 2024).

Department for Education (2020). *Education, health and care plans*. Available at: https://explore-education-statistics.service.gov.uk/find-statistics/education-health-and-care-plans/2022 (Accessed: 14 January 2024).

Miller, S. (2003). *Creating Communication Passports.* Available at: www.communicationpassports.org.uk/creating-passports/ (Accessed 14 January 2024).

Speech and Language UK. (2023). *Listening to Unheard Children: A Shocking Rise in Speech and Language Challenges*. Available at: https://speechandlanguage.org.uk/wp-content/uploads/2024/03/Listening-to-unheard-children-report-FINAL.pdf (Accessed: 22 April 2024).

Thiemann-Bourque, K., Feldmiller, S., Hoffman, L. and Johner, S. (2018). Incorporating a Peer-Mediated Approach Into Speech-Generating Device Intervention: Effects on Communication of Preschoolers With Autism Spectrum Disorder. *Journal of Speech, Language, and Hearing Research*, 61(8), pp. 2045–2061.

5 What We Already Know

This chapter will examine some of the research around Augmentative and Alternative Communication (AAC) abandonment and what barriers educators are currently facing for successful implementation of aided language/AAC in the classroom, so steps can be made to overcome those identified barriers.

It may feel like climbing Everest when trying to support your learners with AAC and aided language in the classroom. Even more so if there is a desire for voice output which then pushes you into the need for electronic AAC. This can mean a battle to seek funding and an ongoing concern around maintenance of the device. Then there is the next big concern: What if the AAC system is abandoned by the user?

What the Research Says

At this point it would be useful for us to look at previous research to highlight factors which have been identified as barriers to successful implementation of AAC. By looking at some of the possible barriers you might face, it allows you to plan how to lower the risk of abandonment and promote successful implementation.

Johnson et al. (2006) conducted a study looking at reasons for AAC device abandonment. Below are the top 20 reasons they identified for AAC device abandonment.

1. Communication partners believe they can understand the person who uses AAC without her or him using the AAC system.
2. Partners do not provide sufficient opportunities for the person to use AAC system to engage in conversations.
3. No need or opportunity to use the AAC system.
4. Lack of motivation on the part of communication partners.
5. User prefers to use other, simpler, means of communication.
6. Professionals who work with the AAC user are not trained to operate and/or program the system.
7. Vocabulary/messages do not meet individualised daily living needs.
8. No time for follow-up training.
9. No time for programming/preparation of materials.
10. No time for team collaboration.
11. User is more independent with unaided communication.
12. No support from family members.
13. Vocabulary/messages are not serving a variety of communicative functions (e.g., requests, protests, comments, narratives, jokes, topic management).
14. System is too difficult to use (i.e., the reward does not justify the means).
15. The family is not trained to operate and/or program the system.
16. Lack of motivation on the part of the user.
17. Communication partners do not model system for the user.
18. Little time for system upkeep.
19. Little time for follow-up training of user and partners.
20. Little time for collaboration with new team members in new location.

Knowing this, it would be useful to think about current practice in education settings and consider where we see common themes which are reflected in research. Once we can identify possible barriers then we can look at how we can support effective implementation of AAC for our learners.

In October 2022 the authors conducted a small survey of educators looking at the use of AAC in schools to try and identify any key themes around barriers to success. It was useful to have the viewpoints of educators who were facing these challenges on a day-to-day basis in the English education system. So far, this book has focused on sharing tips and suggestions around AAC implementation and aided language in the classroom environment. However, we know that life is not always perfect, and challenges are likely to occur. By trying to identify what these challenges may be, we can look at ways to negate them and reduce the risk of abandonment of the AAC provided.

The questionnaire was filled in by 44 educators from a variety of roles in schools. The majority were teachers (including some SENCOs) and teaching/learning support assistants. Most participants were school based, with a greater proportion of those being staff working within specialist settings, where we would typically expect there to be a higher volume of learners with speech, language and communication needs (SLCNs).

The SEND Review in 2022 showed an increase in learners identified as requiring SEN support or Education Health Care Plans (EHCP) with a primary need of speech, language and communication needs identified, and this was reflected in the survey sample with 40 of the 44 participants confirming that they worked with learners who had SLCN. This probably does not come as a shock to you if you are a current classroom practitioner. The increased volume of learners presenting with SLCN does, however, highlight the need for initial teacher training in this area, so educators can confidently support implementation of tools such as aided language and AAC.

> **Discussion Point!**
>
> - Did you have any training on aided language or AAC in your training for your current role?
> - What training would have been useful for you to have had?
> - If you have identified what knowledge you would have liked to have gained prior to working with learners with Speech, Language and Communication Needs (SLCN), write it down now.
> - Could there be an opportunity for peer learning with colleagues within your staff meeting structure?

The most Common Types of Speech, Language and Communication Needs

Identifying the needs of the learner was also explored with participants who demonstrated that they supported learners with a range of SLCN. It would be useful for us to breakdown some of the more common types of needs that the educators supported, as you will likely find yourself working with learners with a similar range of needs.

- Problems with producing speech: These are the learners who may benefit from aided language to augment their natural speech and cue their communication partners into what they are verbally offering.
- Problems understanding language: These are the learners who benefit from aided language input to help them learn language. Aided language has a greater permanence as it doesn't immediately disappear, like spoken language does. An educator can point to a symbol for a longer duration allowing learners more processing time to learn the language.
- Problems using language (word finding skills): These are the learners who need us to model aided language on different communicative functions. They need educators to model that breadth of aided language and see the language choices in front of them to support with skills such as word finding.
- Problems interacting with others: These are the learners who need that explicit instruction in the different reasons why people communicate with each other. For example, 'I'm telling you something. Imogen, I loved your dance in the show.' These learners often even need the most foundational level of support, even around understanding that they need to have another person to communicate with.

The Royal College of Speech and Language Therapists (RCSLT)
This wide range of needs identified, highlights the level of training that educators are likely to need to effectively implement aided language and AAC.

How is Speech and Language Therapy Delivered?

As identified previously in this book, we know that educators are currently seeing a reduction in the amount of access to speech and language therapy in school environments. Participants helped us to gather a snapshot of what type of support educators are currently receiving around speech and language therapy for their learners.

Half of the participants experienced speech and language therapists taking their learners away from the classroom environment to provide therapy. Although it will be appropriate that some therapy is carried out in isolation, it is also key to remember that educators can only implement support strategies if they know how to support learners and can see how it fits into the daily classroom routine. If therapy is always done in isolation away from the class team and class environment, it makes it difficult for educators to have successful implementation of therapy in the classroom. Strong multi-disciplinary teams of educators and speech and language therapists work together in the classroom environment. This means that implementation support strategies can be shared. Consequently, the learner will then have support strategies in place for all the time that they are in the school environment.

Confusion Around Terminology

In both education and health there is a staggering amount of terminology that people presume everyone just knows. We know that often people struggle with terminology, which can lead to confusion and reluctance to get involved. The term Augmentative, Alternative Communication (AAC) is used when referring to a communication system a learner uses. That AAC may also include the use of aided language – a language whereby we assign meaning to something external to our bodies, for example a symbol. When conducting the questionnaire, there was a need to identify whether educators in the sample were familiar with the acronym AAC. If not, this would identify that either the terminology needs to be simplified so it's accessible for all, or training and support should be made available. This will enable all educators to have that shared language and understanding. It was the case that a quarter of the educators involved had not heard of the term AAC.

That is not to say that educators were not supporting implementation of AAC and aided language in the classroom. Many of the participants were using aided language and key word signing in the classroom to aid receptive language, as you can see from the support strategies that the educators were currently using in class (Figure 5.1). This again highlights the need for a common language which spans across health, education and social care.

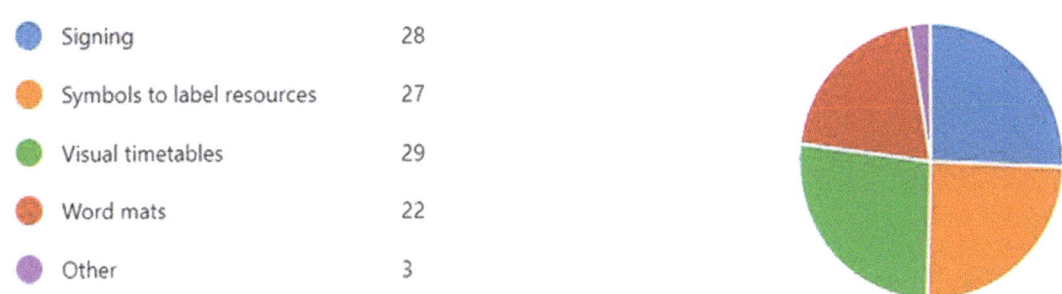

Figure 5.1 This image shows a colourful pie chart.
Source: Created by the author.

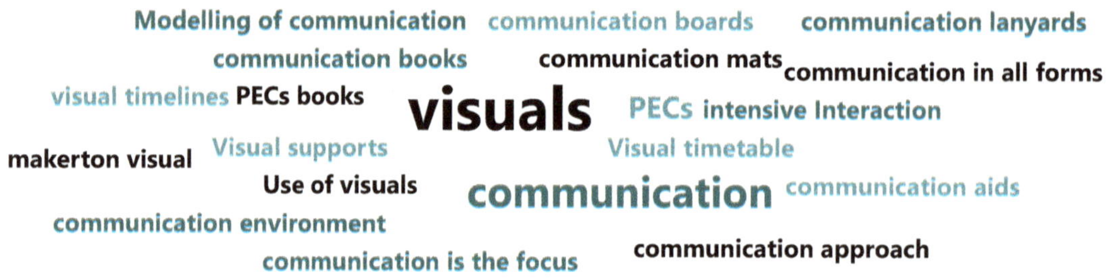

Modelling of communication communication boards communication lanyards
communication books communication mats communication in all forms
visual timelines PECs books **visuals** PECs intensive Interaction
makerton visual Visual supports Visual timetable
Use of visuals communication communication aids
communication environment
communication is the focus communication approach

Figure 5.2 This image shows a word cloud with the word visuals in the middle.

Source: Created by the author.

Resources used in Schools

It may be useful here to have a look at some of the resources that participants in the survey were currently using to support their learners with speech, language and communication needs in class (Figure 5.2).

> **Discussion Point!**
>
> - Have a look at the word *wall*.
> - Are you familiar with these types of resources? If not maybe take some time now to research examples from other educators.
> - Could any of these resources be useful to a learner in your classroom?
> - What language would you have on them for your learner?
> - How could these resources support language development for your learner?

Training

Training around aided language and AAC was also highlighted through the survey. Many of the educators said that any training they had received was in-house or through webinars of companies that make electronic AAC devices. It was interesting to see that no formal qualifications were listed, such as the SENCo qualification or initial teacher training. There was also no mention of any university level qualifications within this sample of educators. We find this reflective of the small amount of qualified training tailored to educators around aided language/AAC. Suppliers such as Liberator, Tobii Dynavox, Assistiveware and Smartbox all have a wide range of training and support available around the AAC they provide. Independent charities such as Communication Matters, Ace Centre and Call Scotland have a wealth of support. This is a good place to start, looking for information and training to upskill yourself in different types of AAC and how to support the implementation of AAC with your learners.

The aim of the survey was to try to take a snapshot image of current practice of both the educators and the more general education system in England when looking at aided language/AAC in the classroom. At the start of the chapter, we looked at the research by Johnson et al. (2006) around AAC device abandonment. The questions asked focused on identifying barriers that the educators were currently facing whilst trying to support their learners with Speech, Language and Communication Needs. Below are some of the key themes that the educators identified when trying to implement the use of aided language/AAC for their learners.

Financial Barriers to Implementation of AAC

Answers shared by participants highlighted issues such as funding, administration for securing funding, the cost of high tech AAC and the cost of repairs of those devices once purchased.

Another participant highlighted that they were successful in getting charity funding for a learner's electronic AAC. The financial barrier they faced happened when the device needed to be repaired. This highlights that there needs to be local AAC services commissioned, which would not only provide, but maintain, a learner's AAC system. A similar national service to this does exist and is called the National Health Service, England Specialised Service for AAC. This service is commissioned to take the top 10 per cent of complex cases of people (of all ages) who need AAC for their face-to-face communication. If you are not aware of this NHS AAC service, please do look it up and familiarise yourself with the eligibility criteria. It could be the case that a learner you are working with is eligible for this fully funded provision. If your learner is not eligible for this pathway, then an alternative funding pathway is required. Some areas do have a local AAC service, though this is not currently a national picture. The learner's speech and language therapist should be able to offer guidance around this. Companies such as Smartbox have lists of charities that would fund electronic AAC and other charities, such as Ace Centre, which could offer guidance around local government-funded pathways.

With electronic AAC often being costly, and no consistent AAC local services in place across England at this current time, it would be worthwhile noting that we can still work on language development with paper-based aided language resources. Lack of funding should not be a barrier to language development. Human communication partners are a lot more forgiving than a computer. A human communication partner knows the context of the communication and can ask for clarification questions to the learner to ensure that they have correctly understood their message. The chapter on teaching symbolic language will support you on your journey with using aided language in the classroom.

Organisational Barriers to Implementation of AAC

Organisational change can be one of the hardest things to achieve. Driving organisational change using a robust AAC policy will be discussed in a later chapter. This will offer tools to help you begin to address organisational barriers you may currently be experiencing. Feedback from the survey (Figure 5.3) conducted identified some key themes that you may be experiencing, too, if you are currently trying to implement the use of aided language or AAC into your school ethos.

As you can see, time, training, and lack of access to a speech and language therapist's support featured consistently in the organisational barriers identified by participants. When asked for more details, participants indicated things like:

> "Staff scared to have a go. Every device is different. Staff slow to get started. Device comes in from home not charged. Staff understand the pupil so don't use the device. Staff expertise and willingness to model constantly."
> "Staff knowledge and confidence."
> "Some staff have a fear of technology."
> "Time with speech therapist. Not enough time for speech therapist to cover all case load."

It is sad to hear that educators feel scared and struggle with confidence in supporting learners with AAC and aided language input. Staff need to be equipped with the skills they need, so not only the learners but the staff themselves experience success. Then they will have the job

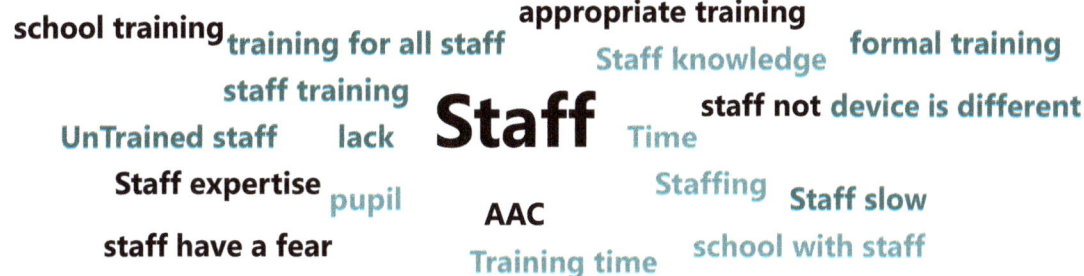

Figure 5.3 This image shows a word cloud with staff in the middle.
Source: Created by the author.

satisfaction of seeing the impact their support has had, rather than knowing there is a problem but not knowing how, or not having the support, to resolve it.

Another organisational barrier which the survey identified was the lack of time. Aided language input is seen as an additional responsibility which places additional time constraints on an already jam-packed curriculum for educators to deliver.

Participants also highlighted that they were not given time to learn about aided language/AAC. They felt that it would be beneficial to be able to have time to practice with the learner's AAC system, away from the live situation of the classroom. Fortunately, many of the AAC suppliers mentioned earlier in the training section of this chapter have options available for partner licences of vocabulary apps, which can then be placed on the school's iPad or computer. This allows educators to develop operational skills away from the live classroom. So, if you are working with a learner who has electronic AAC, please do contact the supplier and see if an additional free partner license is an option.

Technical Barriers to Implementation of AAC

Many of the technical barriers which the educators reported, linked heavily with other factors such as financial and organisational barriers. There were themes such as lack of access to electronic AAC and assistive technology, such as switches for alternative access. They also identified lack of time allowed by organisations for staff to obtain training and familiarise themselves with the technology.

The participants identified some of the more practical issues that everyone has with technology, such as making sure that the device travels with the learner between settings and ensuring that the device has been charged overnight, so it has full battery life to enable functional use for the next day.

Support around troubleshooting was also highlighted as an issue. Who is responsible for maintenance? Who can troubleshoot Wi-Fi and connectivity problems?

> **Discussion Point!**
> - Now, think about any electronic AAC users in your school.
> - If the device breaks, do you know who to seek support from?
> - Is the AAC connected to the Wi-Fi to allow backups of vocabulary edits, or is this done on the home Wi-Fi?
> - Who is responsible for charging electronic AAC? Do school and home have a charger, or do chargers travel between settings with the AAC system?

Lack of Multidisciplinary Working

The final theme that the educators identified was the lack of opportunity to work as a multidisciplinary team with the learner's speech and language therapist (if the learner was on the caseload of a therapist). They expressed opinions around wanting the opportunity for therapists to be in class, modelling best practice to the staff team around how to support implementation of aided language/AAC. It was also identified that having more connected services to share information and support for families would also be useful.

Now we have examined what factors the research tells us leads to abandonment of AAC and we have consulted with a sample of educators working in the English education system, we can identify key themes such as:

- Lack of training in communication partner skills and how to support the setup of the AAC.
- Not enough access to appropriate aided language.
- Not enough time to maintain the AAC system.
- Not enough time to maintain and support the implementation of the AAC device.

- Not enough opportunities to work as a multi-disciplinary team to support the learner,
- Lack of opportunity for the learner to use the device.

> **Discussion Point!**
>
> - Have you experienced similar barriers within your organisation when trying to implement the use of aided language/AAC with a learner?
> - Take some time now to identify any possible barriers and to plan how you are going to overcome them to support your learners.

This chapter has allowed us to delve into some of the research and a snapshot sample of what some educators are experiencing in their roles at this current time. Now that we have identified possible barriers, it leaves us in a stronger position to think of solutions to ensure positive outcomes for those learners who need to use aided language for their face-to-face communication. At this point it is also worth stepping back to the research and looking at what it can tell us around successful implementation of AAC. Johnson et al. (2006) identified the top 19 factors in the long-term success of an AAC user. These factors are listed below:

1. Person who uses AAC system experiences successes.
2. Degree to which the system is valued by the user and partners as a means of communication.
3. System serves a variety of communicative functions.
4. User's physical abilities match system characteristics.
5. Support for the system from the family and user.
6. User is able to access the system accurately and independently.
7. There is a good match between the user's cognitive abilities and the system's characteristics.
8. System is used for communication, not just as a toy or therapy tool.
9. There is support among professionals on the team.
10. Team members (including the family) have time to maintain the system.
11. Team members (including the family) receive continuous support and training with respect to keeping the system operational and making changes.
12. The system is adaptable, flexible and accessible.
13. There is sufficient training for new communication partners in the current setting and during transitions to new settings.
14. Families and the person who uses the system are realistic about the system's capabilities.
15. The user and family members are emotionally ready to accept that a system is necessary.
16. Vocabulary and messages are frequently updated, according to the user's condition, needs, and abilities.
17. The user has a sense of ownership of the system.
18. There is a good level of commitment to advocacy and consistent follow-through by the user and/or partners.
19. The system is portable and so can be used in multiple settings.

Conclusion

All the information shared in this chapter informed you around the complexities and the challenges you may face when using aided language and AAC with your learners. We looked at organisational barriers such as lack of time, funding, training, and collaborative working as part of a multi-disciplinary team.

A good place to start when considering how to overcome these barriers could be to get the environment right. It is important to get the environment right to minimise the risk of abandonment, enabling learners who use aided language/AAC to develop and thrive. This is explored in the next chapter.

Bibliography

Department for Education and Department of Health (2022). SEND Review: Right support Right place Right time. Available at: https://assets.publishing.service.gov.uk/media/624178c68fa8f5277c0168e7/SEND_review_right_support_right_place_right_time_accessible.pdf

Johnson, J.M., Inglebret, E., Jones, C. and Ray, J. (2006). Perspectives of Speech Language Pathologists Regarding Success Versus Abandonment of AAC. *Augmentative and Alternative Communication*, 22(2), pp.85–99. doi: https://doi.org/10.1080/07434610500483588

NHS England (2016). Guidance for commissioning AAC services and equipment. [online] Available at: www.england.nhs.uk/commissioning/wp-content/uploads/sites/12/2016/03/guid-comms-aac.pdf

Royal College of Speech and Language Therapists (no date). *What are speech, language and communication needs?*. Available at: www.rcslt.org/wp-content/uploads/media/Project/RCSLT/rcslt-communication-needs-factsheet.pdf (Accessed: 14 January, 2024).

6 Getting the Environment Right

When considering implementing aided language for learners with Speech Language and Communication Needs (SLCN) within your setting, getting the environment right is crucial. You will often see in classrooms resources to support learners' receptive communication. This may be in the form of visual timetables, labelling resources, and behaviour supports.

Figure 6.1 is an example of a visual schedule for immunisations to support receptive language when explaining to a learner what is happening throughout the day.

Figures 6.2–6.4 show examples of visual supports to help a learner know what equipment is needed for a lesson; steps for end of the school day routine; and a 'now and next' board to show what activity the learner is currently doing and what is coming next.

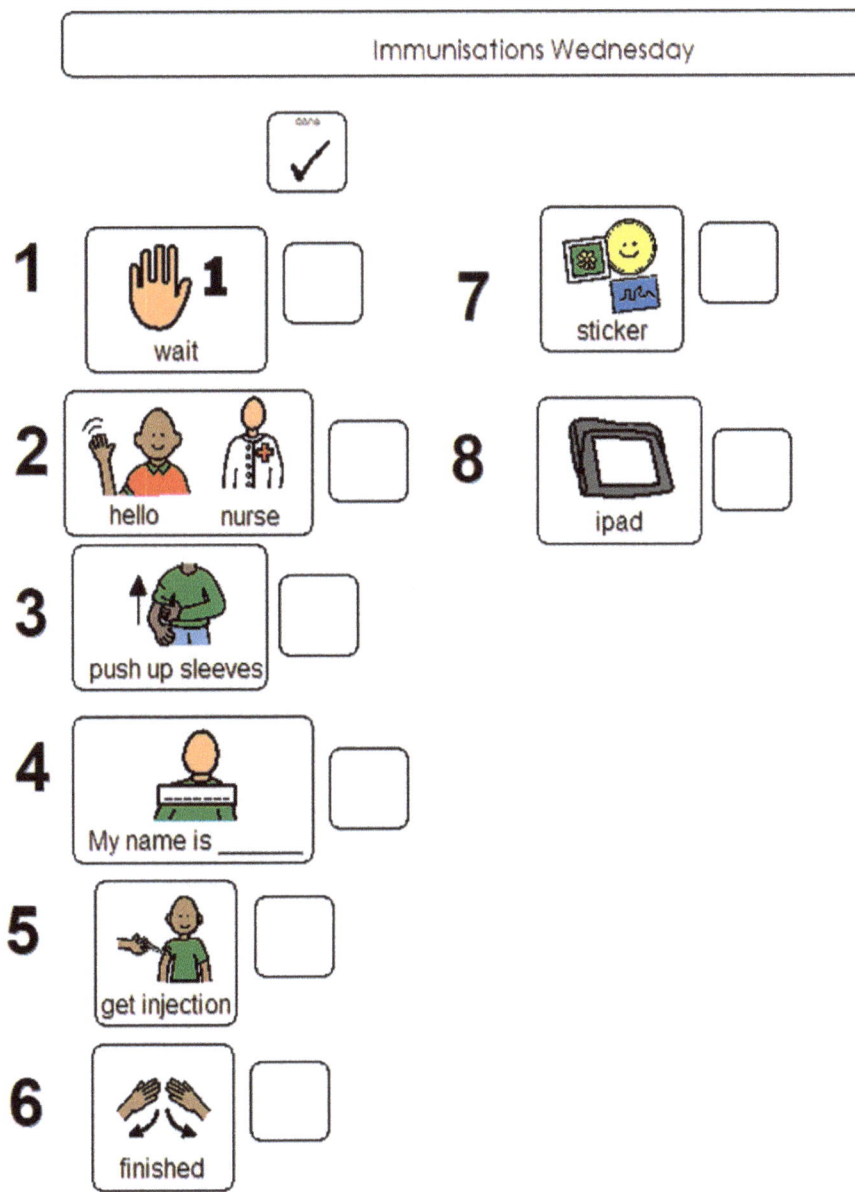

Figure 6.1 This image shows a visual schedule for immunisations.

Source: Created by the author with PCS symbols. PCS and Boardmaker are trademarks of Tobii Dynavox LLC. All rights reserved. Used with permission.

DOI: 10.4324/9781003410836-6

46 *Getting the Environment Right*

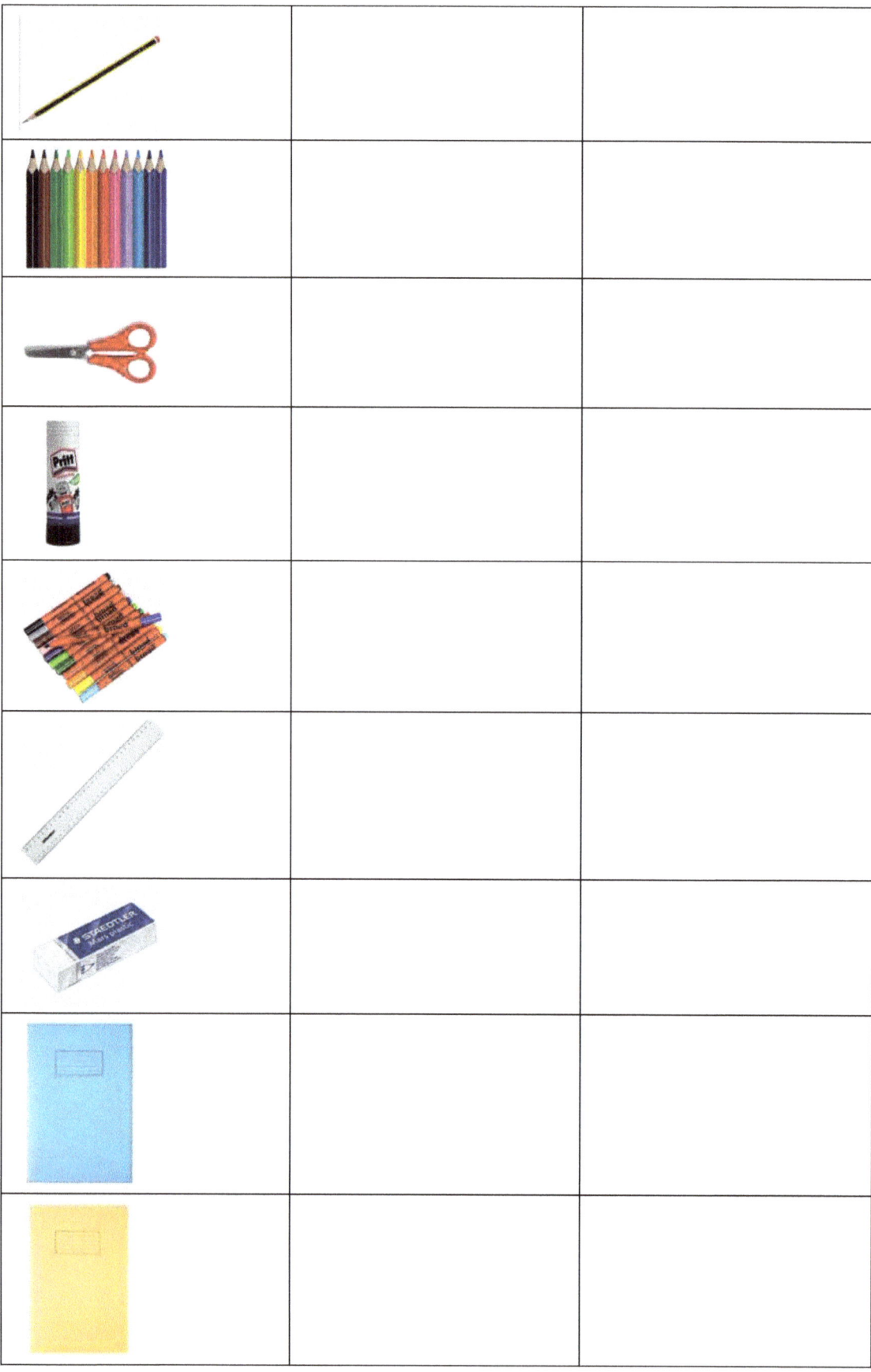

Figure 6.2 This image shows a table labelled 'I need' and with photos of stationary.

Source: Created by the author.

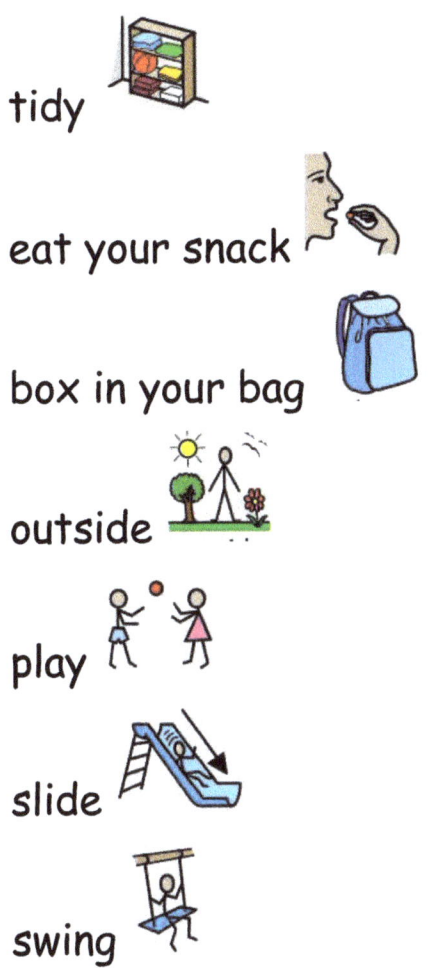

Figure 6.3 This image shows different instructions, with symbols to support.

Source: Created by the author. Widgit Symbols © Widgit Software Ltd 2002–2023 www.widgit.com

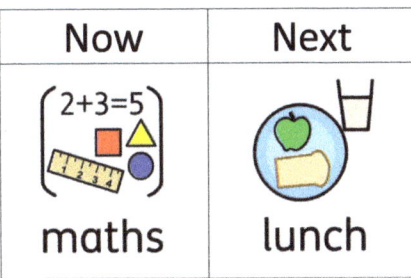

Figure 6.4 This image shows the words now and next with the symbols for maths and lunch.

Source: Widgit Symbols © Widgit Software Ltd 2002–2023 www.widgit.com

These types of support enable learners to better understand the world around them; however, they are not tools to support expressive communication due to the limited vocabulary that they offer.

There are many resources that can be implemented within your classroom environment and beyond to support the development of a learner's expressive language, enabling them to say what they want to say, when they want to say it (Porter, 2018).

The integration of these resources will support learners with Speech Language and Communication Needs. They could also benefit learners within the rest of the class, as aided language, for example, a graphic symbol does not disappear once said, unlike verbal speech. This allows learners additional processing time when exposed to the word. Having aided language resources available in the classroom for all learners to access, will facilitate an increase in social interactions between learners with SLCN and their peers, making them feel accepted within the setting, thus increasing their self-esteem and confidence.

It is crucial these aided language resources within the environment are utilised effectively to support the development of expressive language, as using these aided language resources is a skill that needs to be taught. Another danger zone is that these aided language resources end up being used as curriculum tools. This runs the risk of aided language resources becoming used to simply answer questions, rather than truly supporting learners in working towards the goal of spontaneously initiating conversation on a broad range of topics.

Practical examples are shown within this chapter which you can adapt to use within your setting.

Most expressive language resources can be integrated into your classroom practice without the need for expensive electronic equipment. Some of the examples included can be printed off and used as they are, others require the use of symbol generating software, such as Communicate in Print and Boardmaker. This will enable the production of bespoke examples to be used within your setting, for example aided language resources which are bespoke to a learner's interests and motivators. This will enable greater success in implementation as they will more likely give the learner access to language around topics which are motivating to them, rather than generic examples.

Many schools have access to symbol generating software, however, if you find yourself without access to this software within your setting, it may be worth considering asking if other schools within your local authority, such as your local specialist school, can give you access to theirs. With an increased number of learners with speech, language and communication needs being educated in mainstream settings, educators are having to implement strategies which they have previously not been familiar with to best support the language development for these learners. This is particularly true for learners working at SEN Support level. The number of learners entering the education system with concerning oral language skills is on the rise (Massonnié, Llaurado, Sumner and Dockrell, 2022), causing teachers and school staff to need to adapt their practice to effectively support those learners. Early identification of learners with Speech Language and Communication Needs is crucial to ensure the gap does not widen in terms of their language development and access to the curriculum. Many areas can have access to early intervention teams prior to starting school, including access to preschool home visiting educational services for learners with SEND and their families, however, this is not consistent nationally, causing many children to fall through the gaps.

Within Early Years settings the use of aided language resources can be successfully implemented to support all learners, as all learners are developing their language skills. Due to the structure within Early Years settings, with a focus on learning through play, aided language can be incorporated into the different activities within the classroom. Examples of these will be discussed as you progress through this chapter.

Unlike secondary education, primary education has the resources and skills to be a more inclusive environment for those with SLCN, as these are typically smaller settings with consistent teachers for all lessons, rather than different teachers for each subject, which enables continuity in access to aided language resources to facilitate expressive language, as learners are generally based in one classroom and have access to familiar communication partners. As learners transition to secondary school, this provision often alters.

Aided Language Displays (ALD)

Aided Language Displays (also known as communication and symbol charts) have real power in supporting learners with Speech Language and Communication Needs. These allow Aided Language Stimulation (also known as Aided Language Input). This strategy allows the communication partner, in this instance classroom staff, to model the use of aided language. Modelling this for the learner is fundamental to the effective implementation of aided language. This means the communication partner pointing to key word graphic symbols on the aided language display as they speak. Speaking aloud whilst pointing to the symbols, provides auditory and visual feedback for learners and helps the learner to attribute meaning to the selected symbols, for language development. The process of modelling will be discussed in greater detail in subsequent chapters of this book.

Aided Language Displays are arranged in grid formats. They are generally arranged to enable the sequencing of words to promote sentence production, as opposed to using these aided language displays at a single word level. The aided language displays are arranged left to right, mimicking sentence structure within the English language, with access to core vocabulary on

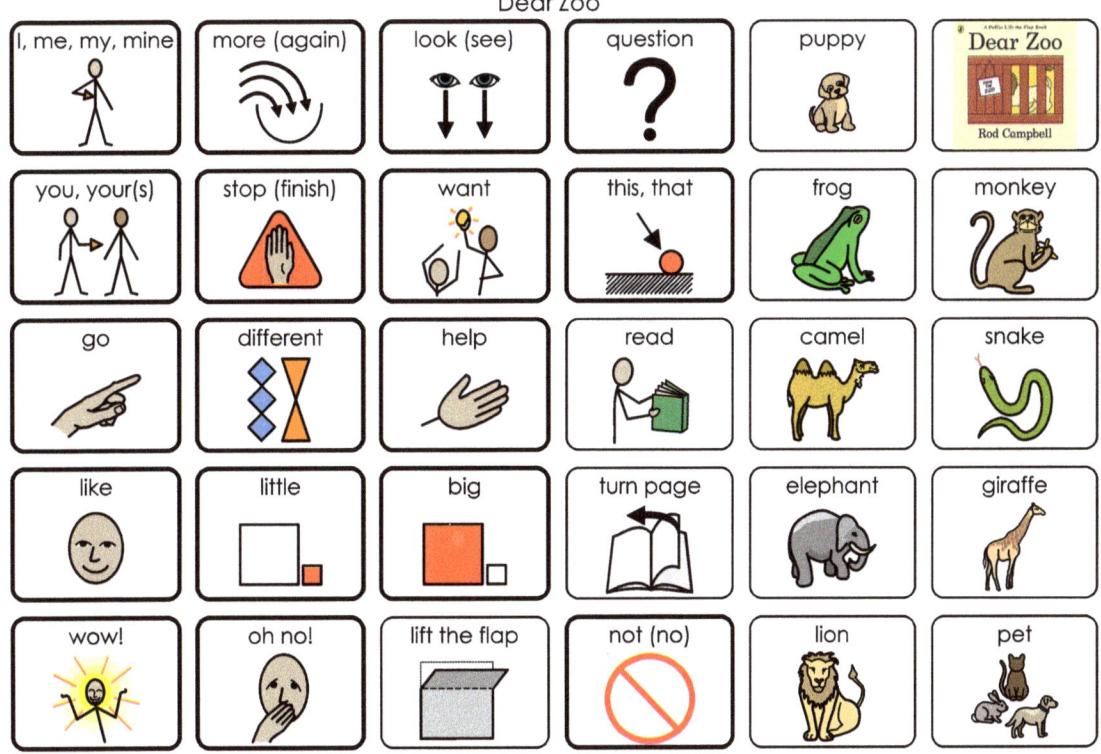

Figure 6.5 Image of 30 symbols with the title *Dear Zoo*.

Source: Created by the Ace Centre https://acecentre.org.uk/resources

the left, and fringe (topic) vocabulary on the right. Here is an example of an Aided Language Display.

This aided language display (Figure 6.5) enables the learner to create a range of sentences in relation to the popular children's book *Dear Zoo*. The variety in the core vocabulary available enables the creation of a diverse range of sentences. Examples of sentences are included below:

- I want turn page
- I like camel
- Oh no! Big elephant
- I see lion
- You help lift the flap
- You read
- Wow! Look that puppy
- Turn the page

> **Discussion Point!**
>
> - Think of other books you are reading with your class.
> - What vocabulary do you feel would be important to have on the aided language display?
> - What sentences would your learners be able to create?

As you can see with these examples, keywords have been picked out from the aided language display rather than always focusing on creating fully grammatically correct sentences. One example of this being 'Look that puppy'. This being grammatically correct would be 'Look *AT* that puppy'. The *at* has been missed out of the sentence. Although you will model by pointing to the symbols, verbally you would include the *at* within your spoken sentence.

This aided language display would support learners with SLCN, but can also be used as a whole class resource, supporting all learners within the classroom environment, particularly

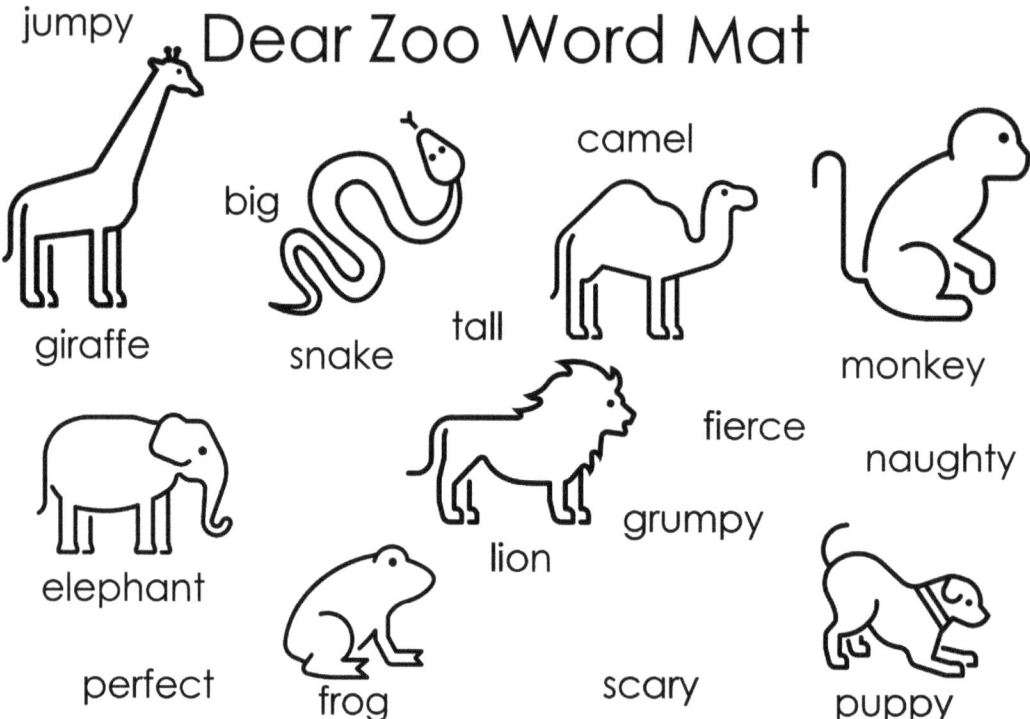

Figure 6.6 This image shows pictures of zoo animals surrounded by words.

Source: Created by the author, adapted from Twinkl.co.uk.

within an Early Years and Key Stage One setting where learners are focusing on sentence construction and may benefit from the visual support. This makes for a more inclusive environment which supports all learners with the same aided language resources.

You will often see word mats used within Early Years and Key Stage One settings. This one links to the story *Dear Zoo*.

This word mat (Figure 6.6) enables Literacy support, predominantly spelling support for learners. This includes both nouns and adjectives to enable a bank of words to be used to write about the story. Examples of sentences include:

- Big elephant
- Tall giraffe
- Perfect puppy

This resource lends itself to combining adjectives and nouns, however, this does not provide the breadth of sentence production that can be seen on Aided Language Displays. This slight change in focus, enables these aided language resources to be used as expressive language supports, which can have a noticeable positive impact on learners with Speech Language and Communication Needs, as they now have access to a language with which they can express themselves.

Aided language displays are cross curricular resources for expressive communication. They are not a curriculum tool for subject-specific learning, for example, not a word mat for sole use in a literacy lesson to support spelling.

Use of Context-specific Aided Language Displays

Aided language displays typically include language around one topic. Therefore, it is important to have a selection of aided language displays which offers expressive language on the full breadth of activities which a learner engages in throughout their day. With many aided language displays in the school environment, learners are immersed in aided language which supports the development of using aided language for expression for those learners with speech, language and communication needs.

Many examples of context-specific aided language displays are available, including some of the examples shown next. Figures 6.7 and 6.8 are two examples which can be used in two distinct different contexts, and a different number of symbols per page.

This aided language display supports playing with cars and can be integrated successfully into both the classroom and home environments. This aided language display could be placed in a box of cars so that it is easily available to support expressive language when playing alongside peers. The example displayed above includes a variety of word forms, enabling a large array of sentences to be produced with just 28 symbols per page. This supports language development beyond the use of single words, as can be seen from the expressive language selected below:

- You drive
- It go fast
- It go slow
- I want stop
- Not drive
- Play again
- You drive lorry, beep beep.
- Stop, crash
- You do that
- Bus drive up

This list of possible sentences includes a range of expressive language – for example, expressing wants, giving instructions, asking for something to stop, commenting and requesting more of an activity, to name a few.

This toileting example shows that aided language can be utilised in all environments, not just to support learning and play, but also personal care. In terms of safeguarding for learners who require personal care, it is important that they have a way of expressing themselves in this environment, due to the personal nature of this activity. Examples of expressive language that could be used are:

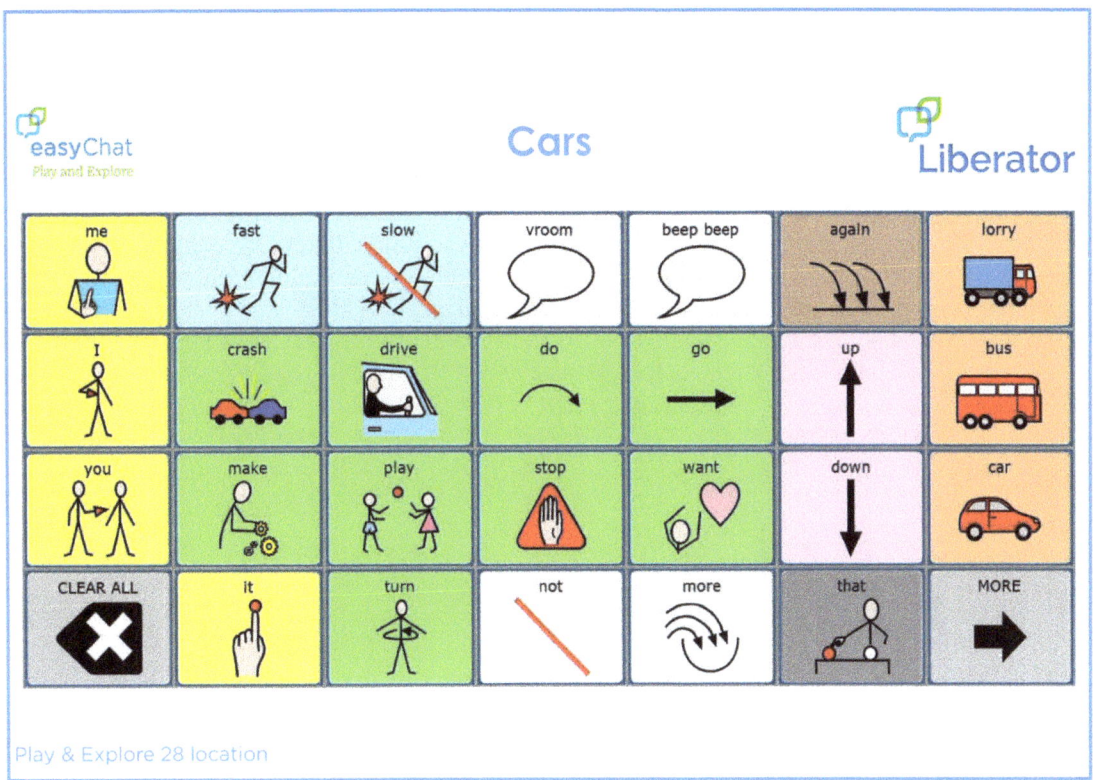

Figure 6.7 This image shows a colourful table with symbols around the topic of cars.

Source: Image courtesy of Liberator Ltd. All rights reserved. Widgit Symbols © Widgit Software Ltd 2002–2023 www.widgit.com

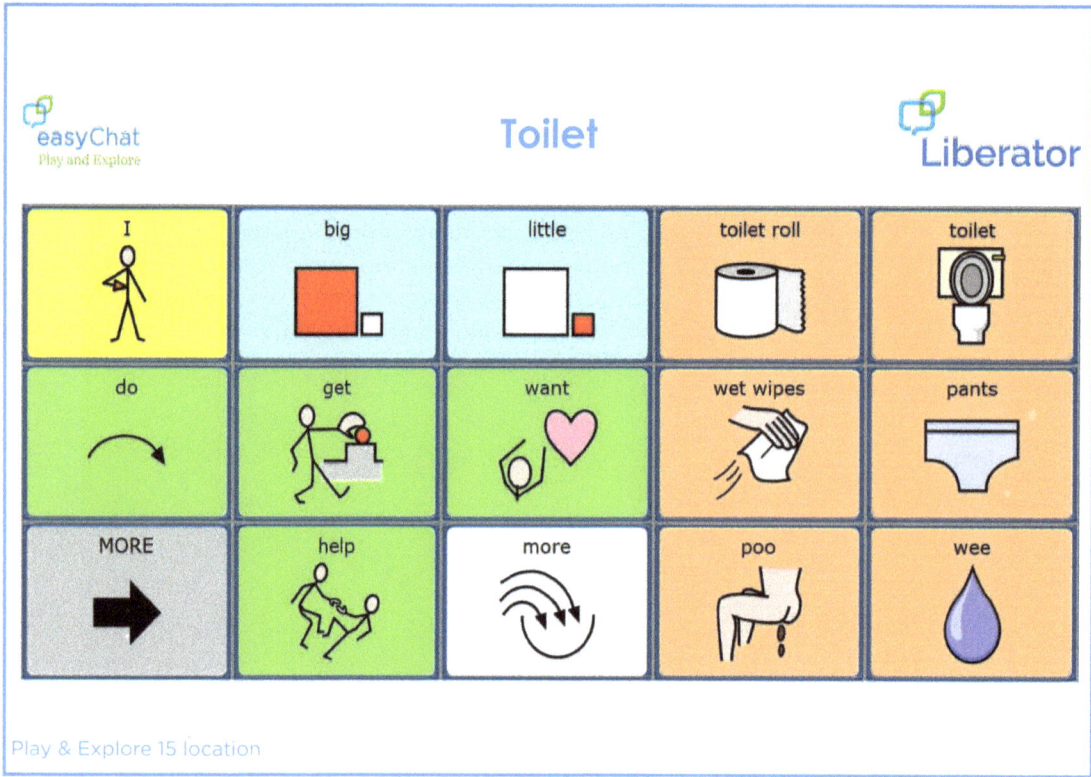

Figure 6.8 This image shows a colourful table with 15 symbols around the topic of toilet.

Source: Image courtesy of Liberator Ltd. All rights reserved. Widgit Symbols © Widgit Software Ltd 2002–2023 www.widgit.com

- I want help
- I do poo
- I do big wee
- More wet wipes
- Get pants
- Help toilet paper
- Help pants little

As you can see from the examples shared, sentences are not always complete and grammatically correct. At this stage where a learner is being introduced to aided language as a tool for expression, there is not the need to focus on grammar as it's more important that a learner can get their message across with the aided language available. It is up to the communication partner to interpret this into a grammatically correct verbal sentence. For example, the learner may use the aided language 'help pants little' and the supporting adult may interpret this as, 'the pants are too small'. Likewise, at this stage of aided language development for expressive language, we would not expect learners to use the correct tense. Once again that would be up to the communication partner to interpret within the context of the conversation. For example, the learner may use the aided language, 'I do big wee', and the supporting adult may interpret this as, 'I did a big wee'.

On a Larger Scale

Aided Language Displays can also be displayed on a much larger scale within learning environments. These could be posters, dynamic aided displays of vocabulary packages on the classroom interactive whiteboard, or playground boards and banners.

Figure 6.9 shows an example of an aided language display poster from the home page of the Easy Chat vocabulary package from Liberator placed below the classroom's interactive whiteboard. This aided language display enables modelling of core vocabulary irrespective of the

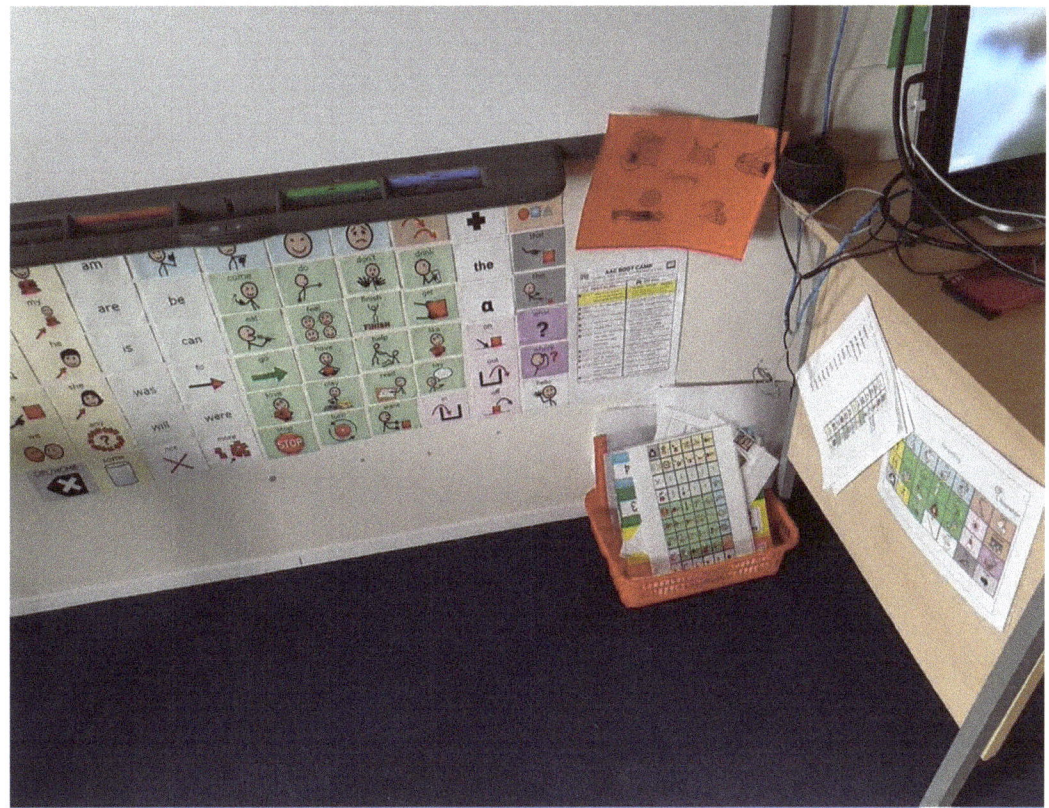

Figure 6.9 This image shows an interactive whiteboard with a table below and colourful symbols.

Source: Photographed by the author.

context of the lesson. The symbols displayed represent a range of expressive language, which can be used irrespective of the learning activity.

Examples of potential sentences include:

- I feel happy
- It finish
- Where you go
- You come in
- It is bad
- She help read
- Don't stop, want play more
- Not like

Figure 6.10 shows an aided language display which has been placed in the outside play area within a school. This increases the opportunities for aided language to be used for expression throughout all environments. Although this example is from a school setting, an increasing number of public parks are now installing aided language displays to support the inclusion of learners with Speech Language and Communication Needs.

The outside aided language display has a range of topic-based fringe vocabulary to choose, for example, ball, bike, scooter; however, it also contains language such as I, where, want, stop, and so forth. This enables the creation of sentences to facilitate the use of a range of expressive language.

Examples of potential sentences include:

- I want scooter
- Your turn/My turn
- Where go
- Ball up/down
- Stop play
- Go toilet

54 *Getting the Environment Right*

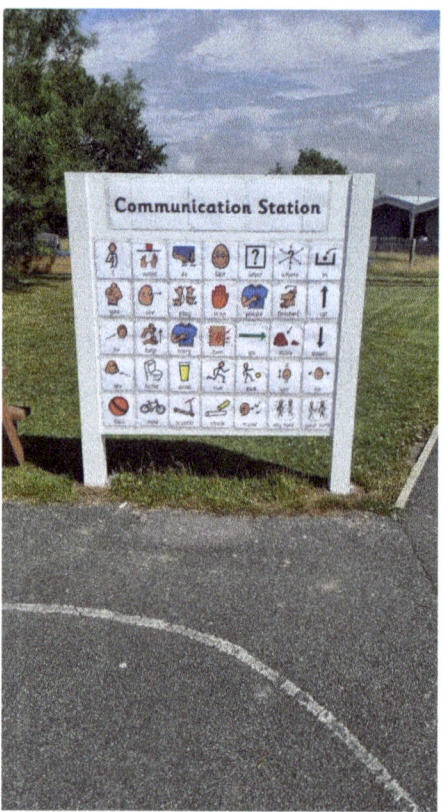

Figure 6.10 This image shows a board with symbols photographed outside.

Source: Photographed by the author, with thanks to Ysol Tir Morfa School.

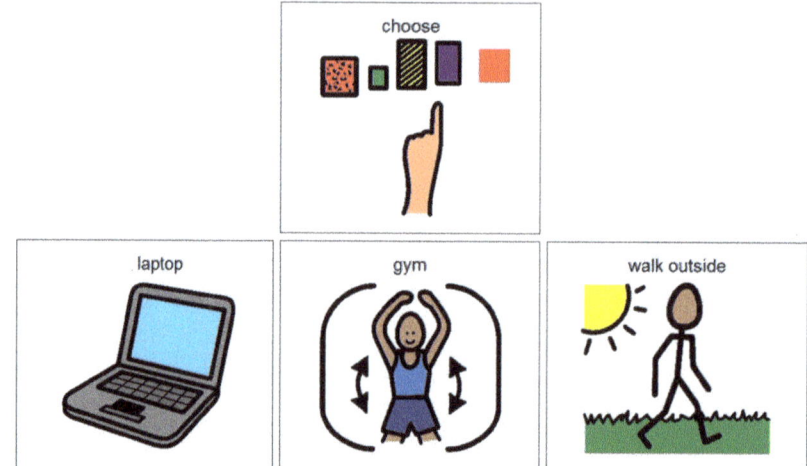

Figure 6.11 This image shows a symbol choice board of 3 leisure activities (laptop, gym and walk outside), created by author using PCS symbols.

Source: PCS and Boardmaker are trademarks of Tobii Dynavox LLC. All rights reserved. Used with permission.

School settings can often be a sheltered environment where learners with SLCN are well accepted by their peers, who have learnt effective communication strategies to facilitate play. However, children within the community who are unfamiliar with the learner may struggle to have effective interactions, which can make the child with SLCN feel isolated. Having access to aided language displays in public playgrounds and parks gives children access to a shared expressive language to chat together and include the child with speech, language and communication needs within play opportunities. Immersing all children in aided language, via the use of aided language displays in all environments, fosters an inclusive society by design. Then no child is left without means to express themselves.

Choice Boards

Choice boards are often utilised within school settings. In contrast to the aided language displays seen above, these generally only include nouns to enable the learner to choose a specific activity/object.

Figure 6.11 is an example of this:

> Compared to previous aided language displays shared within this chapter, what can you say using this choice board?
> Imagine only being offered choices for your expressive communication. How would that make you feel?

Although choice boards give learners a vehicle to request what they want, for example specific snacks, toys, stories and so forth, choice boards do not allow a range of expressive language as seen in previous aided language displays. Choice boards enable the individual to use a single word, for example *chocolate*; however, they do not have access to vocabulary to express whether they want a chocolate, or they are telling you they have had chocolate, they like chocolate, or they may not like chocolate. All they can say is 'chocolate' forcing communication partners to interpret this single word as a request for chocolate. This can cause frustration for the learner if the communication partner interprets this wrongly. The danger of only requesting will be looked at in more detail in a later chapter.

Smaller Scale

The examples discussed above include a range of aided language on different types of displays, but the use of smaller aided language displays which are more portable can often be useful in enabling the learner with Speech Language and Communication Needs to have quick access to expressive language irrespective of the environment. These smaller-scale aided language displays can take the form of symbol keyrings, which are often worn by staff working alongside the learner. This ensures symbols are always on hand to support the expressive language of that learner. You will find many school staff, particularly within specialist settings, will have these attached to their lanyards. In addition to supporting expressive language, these can also be used by the member of staff to support the learner's receptive language. This can be of particular benefit when a learner is in crisis, in a state of sensory overload, or in situations such as transitions. In these moments some learners may struggle to process the spoken words, meaning their receptive language skills are below their usual level when heightened. Symbols have permanence, meaning that symbols can be used as a visual prompt for the learner. Using the graphic symbol allows attention to be drawn to the key word and shifts focus from the face-to-face interaction which some learners, particularly those with a diagnosis of autism, can find challenging to interpret.

Some school staff, or learners with SLCN, may also have small, aided language displays on lanyards which are easily portable. As these are not subject-specific, with access to a broad range of expressive language, they can be used irrespective of the context to support expressive language for learners with Speech Language and Communication Needs.

Figure 6.12 is an example of one from Liberator.

Apron with Symbols Attached

In some environments, such as Early Years settings, having symbols readily available to support expressive language is key. There are many creative ways to do this. Alongside the use of lanyards and keyrings discussed above, there are many other alternatives.

56 Getting the Environment Right

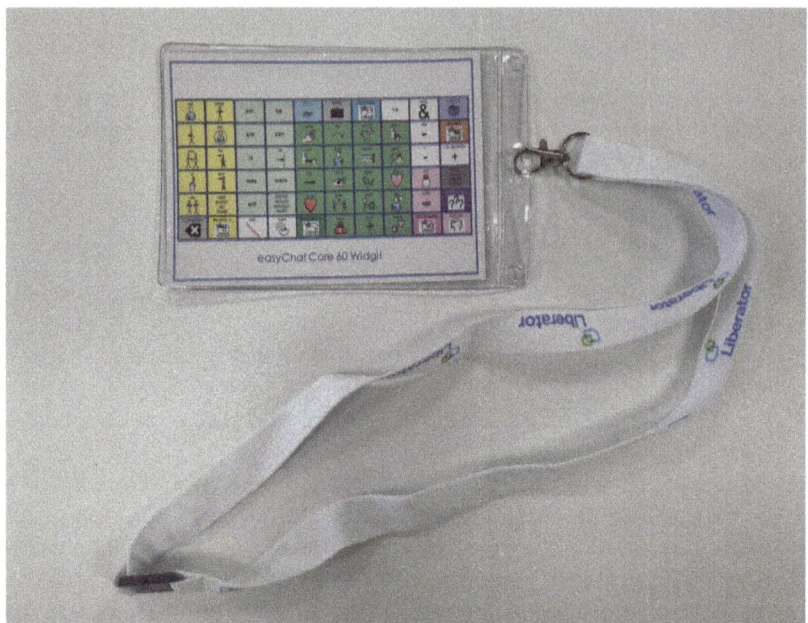

Figure 6.12 This image shows a lanyard with a small, colourful chart with symbols.

Source: Photographed by the author.

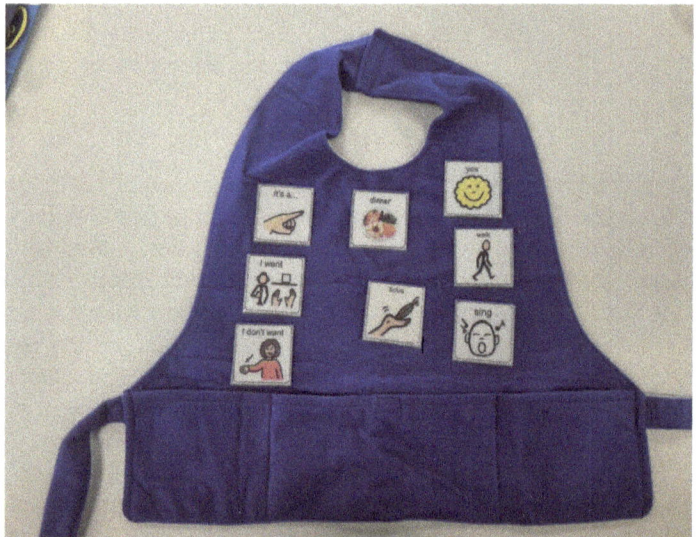

Figure 6.13 This image shows a blue apron with symbols attached.

Source: Photographed by the author.

Having an apron can be handy to store symbols when moving around environments, whilst using these to support a given activity. Young children typically seek out adult interaction, so having the symbols attached to an apron and readily available promotes easy access to that expressive language. The example shown in Figure 6.13, the expressive language relevant to play is placed on the outside of the apron so that it is readily available for learners to select, and for staff to model.

Electronic Alternative, Augmentative Communication (AAC)

Examples discussed so far within this chapter are paper-based resources. These are low cost and easy to implement. You may, however, come across some learners within your class who are using electronic communication aids. It can be challenging to incorporate these into the learning environment in a way that is accessible to all learners. Paper-based resources do not have the functionality to act in a dynamic way, as an electronic AAC device does.

Encouraging staff and peer modelling on a learner's electronic communication aid, can sometimes be challenging. One way around this is by mirroring the learner's vocabulary package onto the classroom's interactive whiteboard. This allows the whole class to see how aided language is organised within the learner's vocabulary package, and how this is used by the learner to express themselves. This can raise the profile of aided language within the classroom and how powerful it can be. This also gives peers a deeper understanding of the learner's electronic communication aid so that they too can talk using aided language and speak the same language as their friend who has speech, language and communication needs. Some companies that supply electronic communication aids also have the option for those around the child to have a partner version of the learner's vocabulary package. This allows the supporting team to have access to the same vocabulary package on a different device, such as the classroom computer.

Conclusion

All the expressive language supports within this chapter provide a language-rich environment for learners. Aided language will become embedded in the practice of staff within the classroom, alongside the power of peer modelling, as discussed within this chapter. Peer modelling can often be overlooked when supporting learners with Speech Language and Communication Needs, however, this can have a huge positive impact on the development of the learner's expressive language. The use of symbolic language and strategy of modelling will be covered in greater depth in the following chapters.

This will begin in the next chapter, where symbolic language is discussed further.

Bibliography

Department for Education and Department of Health (2015). *Special Educational Needs and Disability Code of Practice: 0 to 25 Years*. Available at: www.gov.uk/government/publications/send-code-of-practice-0-to-25 (Accessed: 14 January 2024)

Massonnié, J., Llaurado, A., Sumner, E. and Dockrell, J. (2022). Oral Language at School Entry: Dimensionality of Speaking and Listening Skills. *Oxford Review of Education*, 48(6), pp.743–766.

Porter, G. (2018). *Pragmatic Organisation Dynamic Display Communication Books: Introductory Workshop*. Melb: Cerebral Palsy Education Centre.

7 What Is Symbolic Language?

> - Think of your daily routine, how often are you exposed to different symbols? Do you recognise these instantly?
> - Symbols are wherever you go, from the logos of your favourite brands and food, to emojis we used when messaging friends and family.
> - Use your phone to send a message to a friend about what you did over the weekend using just emojis. Will they be able to work out what you did?

It is worthwhile taking the time to stop and think about what we mean when we use the word *symbol*. In its truest sense we are talking about something that represents something else. In the contexts of school, we use symbols such as objects of reference, pictures or words. In the context of this chapter, when the word symbol is used, it will mean a graphic symbol, as shown (Figure 7.1). When you hear educators talking about a learner using symbols, this is generally what they will mean.

When working with a learner with Speech, Language and Communication Needs, using aided language can offer a way for learners to effectively communicate. Aided language can be described as communication modes that require equipment in addition to the learner's body. So, aided language does not include sign language. One type of aided language is to use graphic symbols. These are pictorial symbols with which a learner can express themselves. They are typically for learners who aren't literate yet and give additional meaning to the words they represent.

There are many symbol sets to choose from, and quite often you will be steered by which symbol software your school or multi-academy trust has purchased. If your setting has not purchased a symbol software, then other options to explore are looking for free premade resources from suppliers, or getting in contact with the specialist school within your local authority and asking them if they could support you with access to symbol-generating software.

Symbol-generating software in schools is often used as a tool to create curriculum resources or resources to support understanding, such as a visual timetable for a learner to better understand their daily schedule. By their very nature, these focus heavily on nouns. We need to shift our mindsets to realise that the symbols are aided language and can be used as a tool for language development for learners with SLCN.

When thinking about using symbols as aided language, there are several places you could look for premade resources. Companies such as Liberator, Smartbox and Tobii Dynavox are good places to start looking, but it's worthwhile noting that companies may have a bias toward one symbol set, so if your learner has particular needs, and you want to explore which symbol set may best suit them, then looking at charities such as Ace Centre can give you a more balanced choice of resources. They have a range of downloadable resources on their website which come in a selection of commercial symbol sets and are free to download and personalise.

Many education establishments prefer that only one symbol set is consistently used, and this generally relates to environmental visuals around the school to support receptive language. Examples of this may be visual timetables, behaviour supports, such as now and next cards or social stories and resource labels. Having consistency throughout a school or college means that the majority of learners only have to learn one symbols set throughout their time at the school or college. When thinking about expressive language support for one learner, it should always be needs-led. An example of this is if a learner had a visual impairment where high contrast symbols would give them better visual access, it would not be advised to say that child cannot have that symbol set as it does not match the symbol set adopted by the school. When looking at supporting a learner's communication, it should always be needs-led to that learner, rather than solely governed by which symbol set the school uses, which one is the most cost effective or any other external reasons.

DOI: 10.4324/9781003410836-7

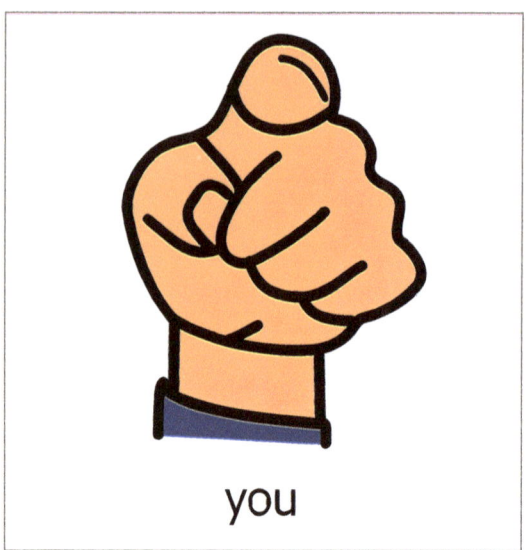

Figure 7.1 A single 'you' symbol.

Source: PCS and Boardmaker are trademarks of Tobii Dynavox LLC. All rights reserved. Used with permission.

What we know from the research is that people learn the symbol sets they are taught. (Sevcik et al., 2018). What is more important is teaching the meaning of the symbols, especially if you feel that a change in symbol set is necessary. As stated, numerous times throughout this book, aided language input/modelling has the biggest impact on language development. Whatever symbol set is deemed best for that learner, it still must be taught. We cannot expect to put communication resources with graphic symbols on, in front of a learner and expect them to just know what they mean. The most important thing to remember when a learner is using symbols is to teach the abstract symbols in the symbol set, as these more complex symbols will often represent the different functions of language, which a learner will need to know if they are to be an effective communicator.

The next part of this chapter will look at a selection of three different symbol sets you may find in the site where you work. There are many similarities between them, but it is also worthwhile to think about some of the subtle differences and therefore which would benefit your learner with SLCN the most.

You can also get these symbol sets in a variety of different languages, and it is always worthwhile exploring options on the company websites, such as Tobii Dynavox and Widgit.

PCS Symbols

The symbols which are now known as PCS symbols (Figure 7.2) were created by speech and language therapist Roxie Johnson. In the 1970s she worked in schools and hospitals and supported children and adults with special needs. It was whilst doing this work that she identified the need for a set of picture symbols to support communication for people with communication difficulties. She formed the company Mayar Johnston with her husband and in 1989 the PCS symbols were incorporated into the Board Maker software. Many schools will refer to this symbol set as Boardmaker symbols. They can be used with different software, such as Grid software by Smart Box.

The PCS symbols are more cartoon-like, and a comparative research of a selection of different symbol sets carried out by Mizuko 1987, found that PCS symbols were transparent, as they were considered to be 'highly suggestive of the referents. As such, their gloss or meaning can be readily guessed by naive viewers.' This is also why educators often miss out doing aided language input/modelling, as learners appear to be using the aided language/AAC because learners can guess the meaning of numerous PCS symbols due to their transparency.

In recent years Tobii Dynavox have developed additions to PCS symbols, such as the thin-line style which is more detailed and realistic than the original PCS symbol set and therefore has greater appeal for adults, teens and children.

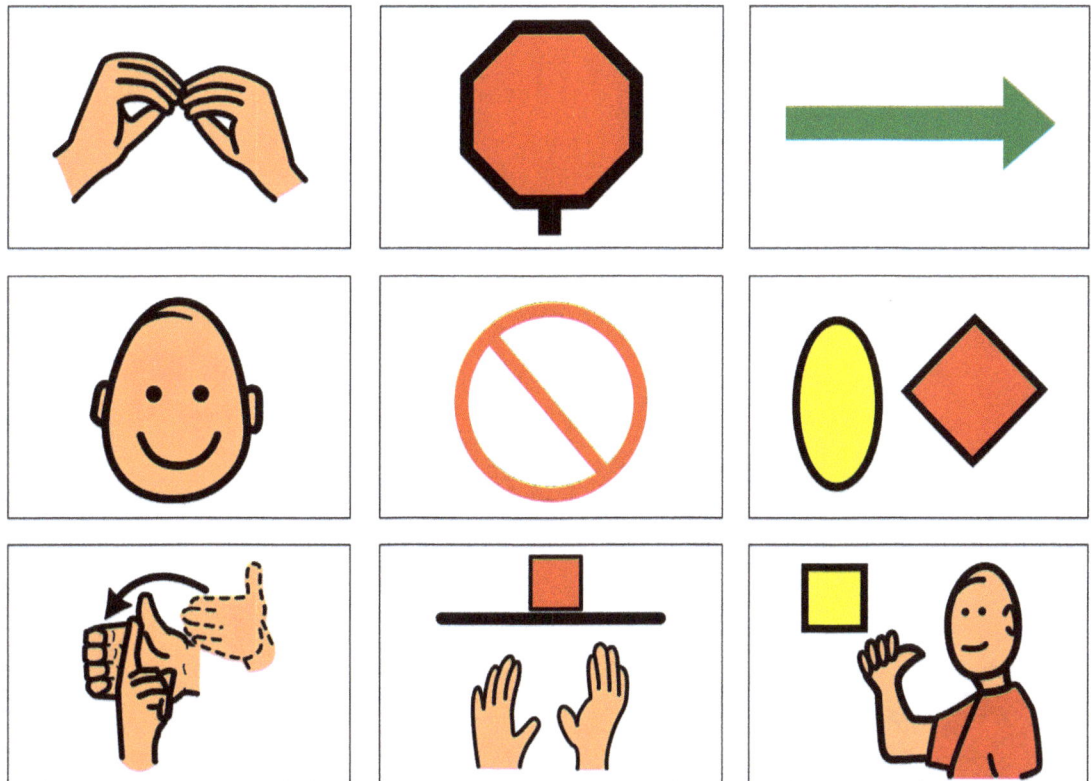

Figure 7.2 A grid of 9 symbols with a with a white background.

Source: PCS and Boardmaker are trademarks of Tobii Dynavox LLC. All rights reserved. Used with permission.

PCS High Contrast

This symbol set, as shown in Figure 7.3, is appropriate to use with learners who have low vision or a visual impairment. It was created collaboratively by the company Tobii Dynavox with the help of Linda Burkhart and Gayle Porter, both of whom drew on experience of working with learners with complex needs. Gayle Porter is the creator of the world-renowned PODD (Pragmatic Organisation of Dynamic Displays) communication system, and if you are working with a child who needs structured support with language development, this is an inclusive system which really scaffolds language development. The high contrast symbols have bold colours to clearly contrast with the black background and minimum detail on the images themselves, to keep them visually simple. They, too, are available in a selection of languages, and it's always worth checking on the Tobii Dynavox website to see the full list of languages supported.

Widgit Symbols

These symbols were initially created in the 1960s and were called Rebus symbols. They were initially created and used in the Peabody Reading Program, in the United States and then further developed by Judy Van Oosterom and Kathleen Devereux to be used in UK schools supporting learners with moderate or severe learning difficulties. Later they were taken over by the software generating company, Widgit. Now they are commonly referred to as Widgit symbols.

The people depicted in this symbol software are generally stick people, which allows them to represent all people, regardless of gender or race. Occasionally, people may be represented fuller than a stick figure to give more information on the person they are representing.

The symbol set follows a schematic structure where additional elements are added to the core concept part of the image to slightly alter its meaning. Figures 7.4 and 7.5 are two examples:

In the study by Mizuko 1987, Rebus symbols alongside PCS symbols, were considered to be the most translucent symbol sets. 'Translucency has been defined as agreement regarding the

Figure 7.3 A grid of 9 symbols with a with a black background.

Source: PCS and Boardmaker are trademarks of Tobii Dynavox LLC. All rights reserved. Used with permission.

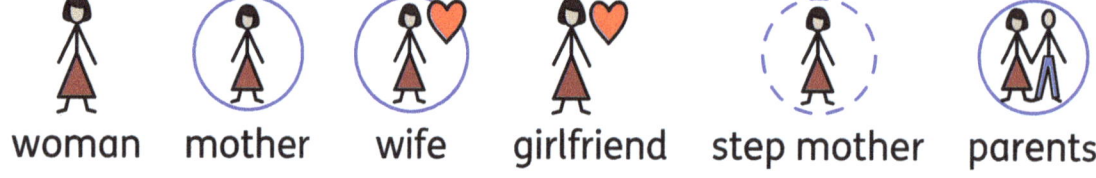

Figure 7.4 A selection of female family symbols.

Source: Adapted from Widgit by the author. Widgit Symbols © Widgit Software Ltd 2002–2023 www.widgit.com

relationships between a symbol and its referent.' (Bellugi and Klima, 1976). In other words Widgit symbols depict concepts well. But, they are not as transparent as PCS symbols which were easier to guess when no instruction had been given.

SymbolStix

SymbolStix like Widgit symbols portray people as stick figures. This once again is to make the people neutral for gender and culture. It is suggested that by removing the detail from the people it gives learners more opportunity to focus on the rest of the information which the symbol is portraying. SymbolStix are one of the newer symbols sets on the market and originated in the United States (Figure 7.6).

Some AAC vocabulary packages offer a choice of symbol sets, so the team around the learner can match what symbol set meets the need of the learner best. Others do not, and those are the considerations a speech and language therapist will assess when introducing AAC with a learner. If you do not have access to a speech and language therapist to do that assessment for your learners and/or you are limited by the resources available to you, for example, the symbol-generating software that the school has purchased, just remember that the most important thing

Buildings

There are two styles of buildings: standard and large buildings. This enables distinction between buildings such as corner shop and supermarket, clinic and hospital.

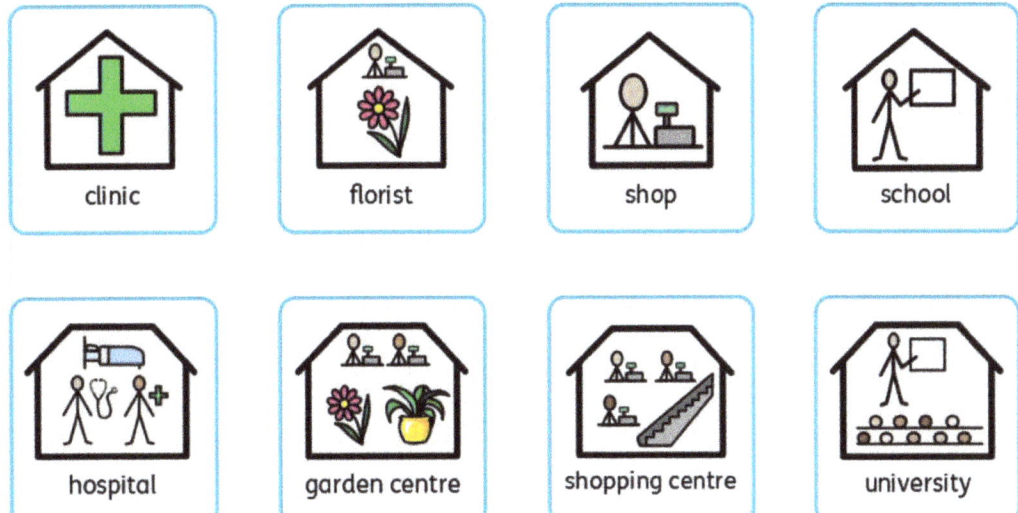

Figure 7.5 Image of 8 symbols of types of buildings.

Source: Created by the author. Widgit Symbols © Widgit Software Ltd 2002–2023 www.widgit.com

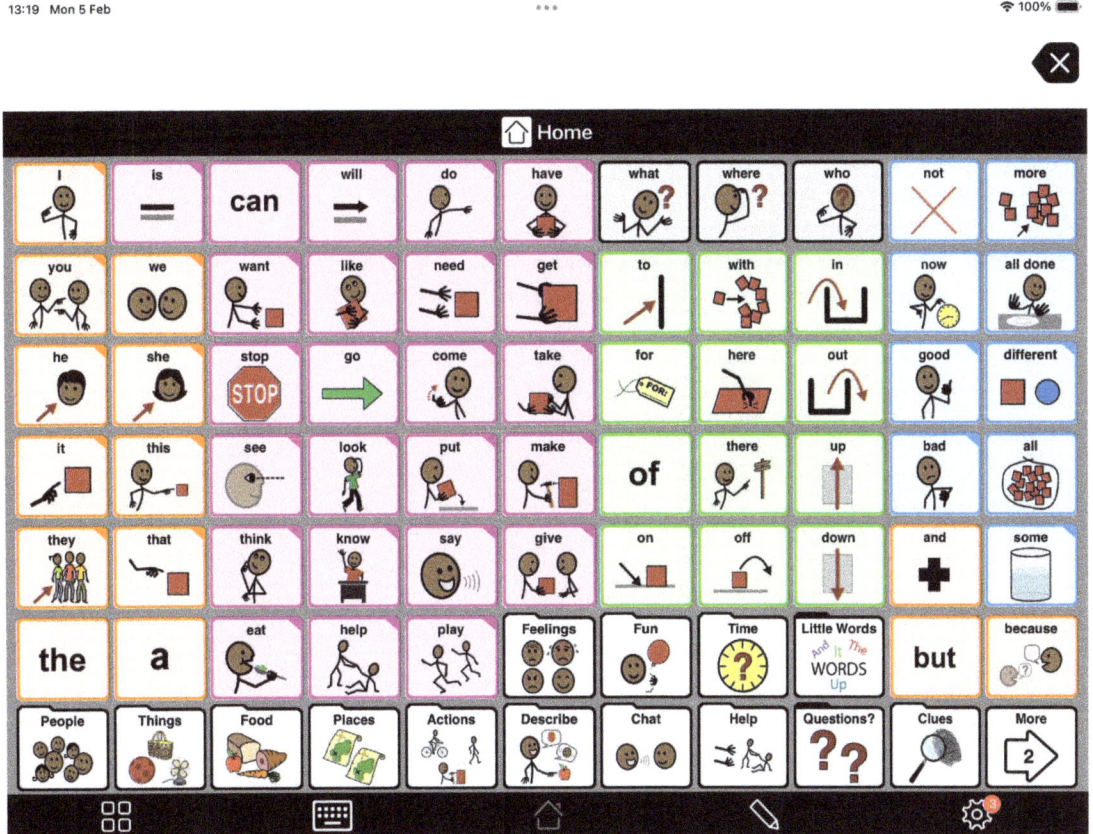

Figure 7.6 Screenshot of a grid of symbols with a black border on the top and bottom.

Source: www.assistiveware.com ©2019 AssistiveWare BV. All rights reserved. Symbols © 2019 SymbolStix, LLC.

is that the learner will learn the symbol set that is taught. It is teaching (aided language input/modelling) which will offer the learner the greatest amount of success to develop language using symbols/aided language.

The PCS, SymbolStix and Widgit symbol sets discussed above are also available to purchase within educational software such as Clicker, which is a literacy support tool. The PCS symbol set is also used in all Microsoft Learning Tools, such as Immersive Reader.

Conclusion

In summary, there is a selection of comprehensive symbol sets to choose from which have enough symbols to support language development for those learners with SLCN who would benefit from using aided language/AAC. PCS symbols are seen as one of the easier guessed symbols sets, as images have a lot of detail and are seen as closer representations to what something may look like in real life. This is probably why many schools have bought into Boardmaker, the symbol-generating software, especially specialist schools where learners may also have learning difficulties. The transparency of the symbols lead to greater success without as much direct teaching/aided language input. Widgit symbols are a carefully thought-out language set where concepts remain consistent throughout, and have additional information added to the core part of the symbol to add additional meaning.

Widgit and SymbolStix both mainly use stick people to allow them to represent across genders and cultures, but again by doing this, learners must understand that the more abstract stick figure represents a person. These symbol sets may require slightly more teaching/aided language input for some learners.

Now we have looked at the different symbol sets available, it is time to consider in the following chapters, how the symbols are to be taught to support learners who use aided language/AAC.

Bibliography

Bellugi, U. and Klima, E.S. (1976). Two Faces of Sign: Iconic and Abstract. *Annals of the New York Academy of Sciences*. doi: https://doi.org/10.1111/j.1749-6632.1976.tb25514.x

Mizuko, M. (1987). Transparency and Ease of Learning of Symbols Represented by Blissymbols, PCS, and Picsyms. *Augmentative and Alternative Communication*, 3(3), pp.129–136. doi: https://doi.org/10.1080/07434618712331274409

Sevcik, R.A., Barton-Hulsey, A., Romski, M. and Hyatt Fonseca, A. (2018). Visual-Graphic Symbol Acquisition in School Age Children with Developmental and Language Delays. *Augmentative and Alternative Communication*, 34(4), pp.265–275. doi: https://doi.org/10.1080/07434618.2018.1522547

8 How Do We Teach Symbolic Language?

The range of different examples of symbolic language have been identified within earlier chapters but, how do we teach this effectively within the classroom environment for learners with Speech, Language and Communication Needs (SLCN)?

Professionals, such as speech and language therapists can support the assessment process, identifying key appropriate features such as which symbol set meets the specific needs of a learner, the most effective way to organise the aided language within an AAC system or aided language displays and making decisions on the appropriateness of paper-based or electronic AAC systems. However, due to current constraints within NHS speech and language therapy services, this support often stops there, requiring school staff to work on implementation of AAC with limited guidance. It is positive for a learner to have an effective communication system in place without having underpinning knowledge regarding how to teach the use of aided language/AAC, there is a high risk of abandonment. You cannot expect a learner to pick up an AAC system and use it effectively for expressive language without any prior teaching.

How to implement a learner's chosen AAC system can often be overwhelming, particularly if the teacher is not familiar with using Alternative and Augmentative Communication (AAC). Teachers can be anxious about getting it right and having to know the ins and outs of the system to support the learner. This can cause an obstacle to be put in place to hinder effective implementation. Staff do not have to have the perfect understanding about the AAC system, but be willing to learn alongside the learner. If the learner can sense that the adult with them is anxious about getting things right, this can have an impact on the learner's willingness to use the system. It is important all staff are on board within the classroom to enable effective implementation of the learner's AAC, otherwise this inconsistency can cause confusion for the learner.

So how do we overcome these challenges and effectively teach symbolic language?

Assigning Meaning

When first considering teaching symbolic language, it is important to know whether the learner has an understanding of what the symbols represent. The symbols, even those that are pictographic, can be abstract for the learner without direct teaching regarding what the individual symbols represent.

> ### Discussion Point!
>
> - Look at this symbol, what do you think it represents?
>
>   ♌
>
> - Can you make a guess based on purely what it looks like?
> - How confident do you feel that you know what it is?
> - How often have you seen this symbol in life?

- How did you find this? It is impossible to understand what it represents without any prior knowledge and understanding, or direct teaching.
- Let's now break this down, imagining you are the learner.
- Look at the first symbol. Visually, without any context this is challenging to identify.
- Now to give some context.

You are taking part in a lesson talking about pets. Does this help at all? Are you able to make any links from what is being verbally discussed and the symbol without this being referred to within the lesson? Can you use it to join in the classroom discussion? Still tricky isn't it!

Now to include those symbols within the context of the lesson.

The lesson has reached the point where the teacher knows that you have a pet snake, however you are unable to share this with her as you do not have a robust AAC system in place and haven't yet learnt the symbol for 'snake'! The teacher points to the picture as she verbally says 'Ah, you have one of these!', but then continues with the lesson without referring to this. Is referring to it just the once, without backing this up with verbal speech, enough for you to understand what the symbol represents?

Now to focus more specifically on the symbol.

Within the lesson your teacher knows that you have a snake. As she discusses this, she points to the symbol and says, 'You have a snake!' Within this lesson she points to it just the once and does not refer to this within the lesson.

Can you recall what the symbol represents?

Now, as your teacher talks about your snake, each time she points to the symbol and says 'snake', ensuring you are focused and attending to where she is pointing. She does this several times within the discussion, breaking down the discussion so it is simpler than it has been previously.

What about now? Have you learnt it yet?

In the final example, the teacher engages in a conversation with you; not only does she point to the symbol several times whilst saying the verbal word 'snake', but she also pauses and leaves space for you to point to and use the snake symbol yourself, without expectation for you to do so.

Can you now recall what the symbol represents? Will you now be able to generalise this skill?

Although you may now have learnt what the symbol represents, by solely doing this within one discrete lesson, can you now use this at home when talking about the snake with your family? Talking to your friends? Talking to staff at the pet shop?

It is so important for this symbol you have now learnt to be used in different environments and contexts.

Breaking down the individual steps shows just how challenging it is for our learners who are using symbolic language to understand what each symbol represents.

There are several strategies used within this example, which you may have noticed helped you in learning what the symbol represented.

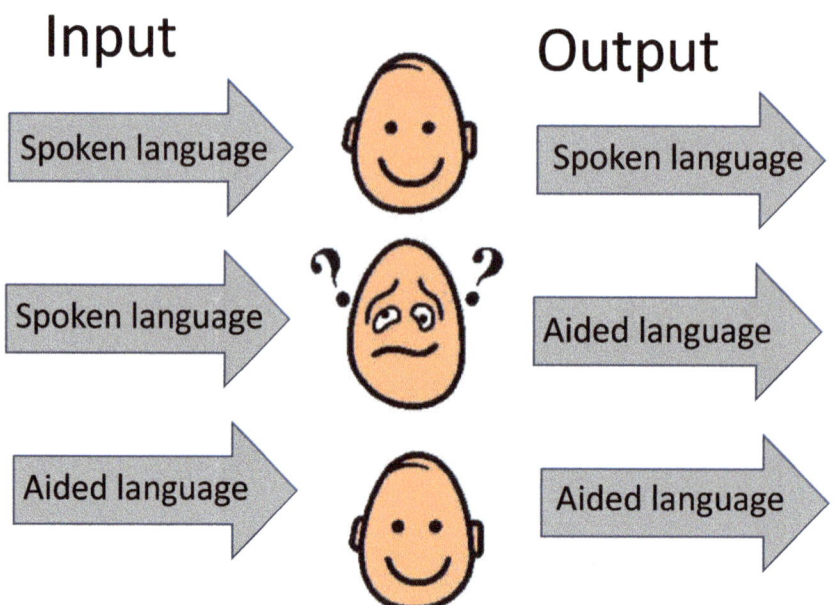

Figure 8.1 This image shows three faces with blue arrows.

Source: Created by author, adapted from Gayle Porter (2004).

First, when talking about your pet snake, the teacher pointed to the symbol itself as they said the word. It is integral if you are teaching a learner who is using aided language – for example in the form of symbolic language – that you also use aided language alongside them, meaning you are speaking the same language.

Typically, learners who use spoken language hear spoken language being used around them and can process this spoken language and are thus able to use spoken language for their expressive communication. For those who use aided language, this becomes more challenging. If solely spoken language is used, the learner can then struggle to translate spoken language into aided language for expressive communication. The ideal is when the communication partner uses aided language alongside the learner, to then enable the learner to use aided language themselves.

Considering the example where the teacher referred to the snake symbol (Figure 8.1) just once, and the conversation then moved on, which proved challenging to retain what the symbol represented and assign meaning. It takes time for learners to understand the meaning and use of symbols effectively, you cannot expect learners to use these symbols when they have only been modelled to them once.

Look again at the example above, where spoken language is the input and output. Now think of a newborn baby. From birth we will use spoken language with them. We will talk to them without expecting any language back. We will immerse them with spoken language until they are around 18 months old, with no expectation of the child speaking. What would have happened if over those 18 months the baby was not spoken to as they were unable to speak themselves? This would have huge implications in terms of the baby's language development. The same is true for using symbols in aided language. We must first attribute meaning to the symbol before expecting the learner to use it independently. This can take time just the same as in the development of spoken language. It can take a significant amount of time modelling before the learner will begin using symbols in aided language themselves, however it is important not to give up and become frustrated that it isn't working.

When working with learners who use symbolic language, it can be tempting to give heavy prompts rather than allowing time for the learner to process information and respond independently. The AAC prompt hierarchy (Figure 8.2) identified healthy and harmful strategies to use with learners who use symbolic language:

When you were imagining the conversation about your pet snake, did the teacher present you with a selection of symbols, such as 'I', 'have', 'a', 'snake', or just the one symbol for 'snake'?

Teachers can often become bogged down feeling they have to find a symbol for each word within a verbal sentence. Using a symbol-based AAC system this can be incredibly challenging, with full sentence production being slow. This can be frustrating for all concerned and overwhelming for the learner. Insisting on full sentence production can slow down communication, causing the learner to give up on communicating their message, which can then also lead to challenging behaviour.

Rather than using symbols to represent every word, instead verbally say the full sentence and only point to key word symbols within the sentence. For example, 'The snake is under the log', you would simply point to the symbols 'snake', 'under' and 'log', whilst verbally saying the full sentence. This then teaches learners the strategy that they do not need to slow down their communication by locating each word in their AAC system, instead communicating in the most efficient way by only selecting key words.

This chapter has discussed modelling using aided language, but what is modelling and how can it be used?

Modelling

Modelling is the term used to describe the strategy of pointing to the words on the learner's AAC system as you speak. This can be used in a variety of different ways and take several forms, some of which are listed below:

1. *Personal modelling*
   This occurs when you use symbolic language each time you interact with the learner. This does not mean finding symbols for each word, instead using available symbols to model a few key words. An example of this could be, 'Hi Peter! Do **you** want to **go** outside **now?**'

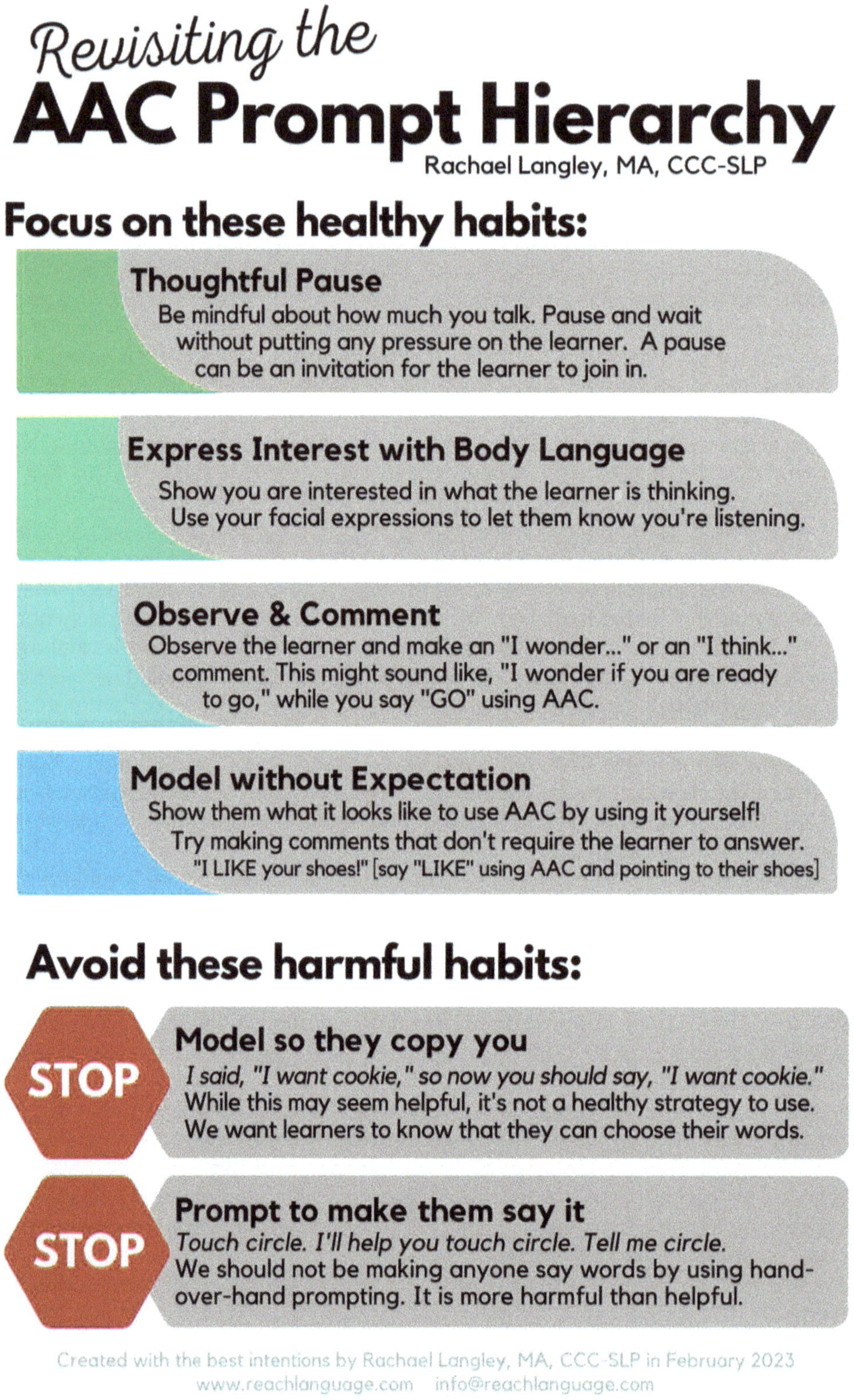

Revisiting the AAC Prompt Hierarchy
Rachael Langley, MA, CCC-SLP

Focus on these healthy habits:

Thoughtful Pause
Be mindful about how much you talk. Pause and wait without putting any pressure on the learner. A pause can be an invitation for the learner to join in.

Express Interest with Body Language
Show you are interested in what the learner is thinking. Use your facial expressions to let them know you're listening.

Observe & Comment
Observe the learner and make an "I wonder..." or an "I think..." comment. This might sound like, "I wonder if you are ready to go," while you say "GO" using AAC.

Model without Expectation
Show them what it looks like to use AAC by using it yourself! Try making comments that don't require the learner to answer. "I LIKE your shoes!" [say "LIKE" using AAC and pointing to their shoes]

Avoid these harmful habits:

STOP — Model so they copy you
I said, "I want cookie," so now you should say, "I want cookie." While this may seem helpful, it's not a healthy strategy to use. We want learners to know that they can choose their words.

STOP — Prompt to make them say it
Touch circle. I'll help you touch circle. Tell me circle. We should not be making anyone say words by using hand-over-hand prompting. It is more harmful than helpful.

Created with the best intentions by Rachael Langley, MA, CCC-SLP in February 2023
www.reachlanguage.com   info@reachlanguage.com

Figure 8.2 This image shows the AAC prompt hierarchy with green boxes and red stop boxes.

Source: Adapted by Rachel Langley, MA, CCC-SLP Speech-Language Pathologist (2015).

2. *Modelling to attribute meaning*

    This is a vital strategy to use with the most complex learners. This enables the communication partner to unpick what it is the learner is communicating in non-verbal, non-formal ways. For example, is the learner expressing excitement? You can acknowledge this and model back 'You seem **happy** today!' This form of modelling requires strong observation skills from the full team supporting the learner and the use of the profiling tools (described in upcoming chapters), to record a learner's pre-intentional and non-formal communication, for

example the Affective Communication Assessment and Pragmatic Profile for People Who Use AAC.
3. *Scaffolding with Modelling*
   This technique can support more able learners, who have an established AAC system in place. This involves adding an additional symbol to the message the learner has expressed to extend their expressive communication. If they respond at a one-word level, you can model back at a two-word level. For example, if the learner selects the symbol '**bubbles**' during a play activity, you can model back 'Do you want **more bubbles?**' by selecting the symbols **'more'** and **'bubbles'**. Similarly, if the learner were to say **'more bubbles'**, you could model back 'Do you **'want' 'more' 'bubbles?'**

Remember, when first starting to model, it can be daunting to do. However, don't be afraid to give it a go! Any modelling is more effective than none, irrespective of your confidence levels. Don't be scared to get started and build up over time, as you become more confident in doing so and it becomes more natural. It will become easier over time.

> **Discussion Point!**
>
> - Consider your different learners. Which forms of modelling do you feel would be most appropriate to use?
> - Think of an activity and how you could model using your chosen form of modelling during this.

Why Is Modelling Important?

Modelling is vital for the learner to become familiar with how to use their AAC system. This includes learning what the symbols represent, but also where to find required symbols and to use these for expressive language. The more you model with a learner, the more experienced and efficient they will become using their AAC system. It is important to model as often as you can! The more the better!

Janice Korsten, cited by Farrall (2014), identified that if learners solely see aided language being modelled to them twice weekly for 20–30 minutes, for example within Speech and Language intervention sessions, it will take 84 years for them to have the same exposure to as much language as an 18-month-old typically has! A child of 18 months has heard 4,380 hours of spoken language before they are even expected to use spoken language.

Benefits of Modelling

Despite staff becoming daunted by the prospect of modelling, this strategy can be simpler to implement than planning structured lessons, as seen in the table below.

Modelling	Structured sessions
More natural – mimics how we actually learn language.	**Very specific** – focusses on teaching specific vocabulary the learner needs to know.
Less pressure – there's no right or wrong answer.	**Teaches** word combinations and grammar.
Less time-consuming – no need for time-tabled teaching sessions	**BUT**
	Time consuming
Less resources required – worked into existing lessons, meaning no bespoke activities need to be planned and resourced.	Requires activity to be **planned and resources** found/made.
	Can be perceived as a **curriculum task** by the learner, rather than communication.

However, both should be used in tandem for the learner to have the greatest chance at using aided language for expressive communication.

Structured Sessions

For these to be used most effectively, they should be planned for in advance. Often these can focus on a particular core word for that day instead of fringe vocabulary, or a given communicative function. This can then be incorporated into activities throughout the day. Post-it notes can often be helpful in these activities in order to plan what you want to focus on.

Some helpful examples of what to consider when planning sessions can be seen in Figures 8.3–8.5, these resources are from the AssistiveWare website, 2023 and Liberators 'Teaching Core Words Across the Day'.

Babbling and Happy Accidents: What are these and Why are they Helpful?

Alongside modelling, there are two further strategies which support learners use of symbolic language: 'babbling' and 'happy accidents'.

Babbling
If you think of a baby in their first year of life, they will 'babble', playing with sounds before speaking proper words. In much the same way, learners will 'babble' using their AAC systems. They will appear to randomly select symbols or press buttons repeatedly on their electronic AAC. This can be viewed as the learner 'playing' with the device, leading to those working around them feeling they are not using the AAC system appropriately and concluding that the learner is not ready to use it. Sadly, in some circumstances electronic AAC (speech-generating devices), can be removed from the learner as they are viewed as just playing with it, rather than using it intentionally, which can cause disruption in class. This can also be viewed as the learner stimming, by pressing the buttons on repeat, enjoying the auditory feedback this produces.

Despite these perceptions, babbling is part of the aided language/AAC learning experience. Whilst doing so, like babies, learners are practicing putting sounds together. This plays a fundamental part in learners understanding the location of vocabulary without the need for modelling. Through going in and out of different pages and folders, they will be able to locate vocabulary. The more they do so, the more they will become familiar with the pathways to find desired vocabulary, especially if the language is motivating for the learner, e.g. names of modes of transport. Over time you will see an increased ability to initiate intentional communication, using the

Function	Core words	Core words with fringe
Requesting	I want, want that, want more, want different	want drink, want to play, I want blue, I want to watch TV
Protesting	stop, not, not that	not yellow, not that toy, stop that music
Commenting/directing	I do it, see me, get, get it, get that, give me that, put it in, take it out,	get the pink one, put your coat on, make a picture, do more jumping, I see the dog
Asking for information	Who? Who go? What? What that? Where? Where go?	What are we doing? Where is mum? Who is going to the park?
Giving opinions	that good, that bad ,like, I like that, I don't like it	I like cake, I don't like snakes, Cats are good, cheese is bad
Tell news	I see, I go, I eat, I saw, I went, I ate	I went to the cinema, We saw daddy, I ate yoghurt for pudding on Friday

Figure 8.3 This image shows a table labelled function, core words and core words with fringe vocabulary.
Source: Created by author, adapted from ©2023 AssistiveWare BV. All rights reserved.

Activity	Core words	Core words with fringe
Cooking	help, need help, like this, not like this, make this, make more, get that, put in there	make biscuits, get some sugar, put milk in, I like chocolate biscuits
Mr Potato Head	put on, take off, need that, need help, looks good	need arms, put on his moustache, take off glasses, looks silly, looks like a fireman
Puzzles	what? where? where goes? look, take out, I do help, need help put in,	what does puzzle make? where dloes this piece go? put dog piece in, I can do with sister
Music	want more, want different, turn on/off/up/down, what next? do it again, like, not like, good, bad	turn on iPad for music, turn on Spotify, I want Taylor Swift, I want to listen to more, No more Hrry Styles, what music do you like?

Figure 8.4 This image shows a table labelled activity, core words and core words with fringe vocabulary.

Source: Created by author, adapted from ©2023 AssistiveWare BV. All rights reserved.

AAC system, and babbling will become less frequent, as seen with babies developing verbal language.

It is important to make sure all staff are on the same page when it comes to babbling, so that staff are aware of the importance of this and the role it plays in the learner becoming familiar with the AAC system, rather than staff perceiving it as an annoying noisy toy! This can also be a stumbling point for parents when the learner first uses the device at home. So having conversations around babbling can be vital.

Happy accidents

'Happy accidents' are also an important tool in supporting a learner in assigning meaning to symbols in their AAC system.

Similar to babbling, learners will randomly locate vocabulary on their device, which appears out of context and irrelevant to the situation. This could easily be dismissed as the learner not understanding the function of the device; however, a rich learning opportunity.

How often with toddlers do you end up having the most random conversations and wonder how you got onto such a random subject? Do you redirect a toddler saying that it isn't relevant to talk about a dragon eating a whale, but is saved by a flying pig? No, you engage in the conversation and step into their world, no matter how unrealistic it becomes!

Happy accidents are much the same. When learners end up making random comments that don't seem relevant, harness these as learning opportunities. Have a discussion around what they have said, however random, as this will support the learner in assigning meaning to enable them to use those symbols in future conversations. This can become great fun! If truly learner-led it can offer the best opportunities to assign meaning to more obscure topic language, which may not have been previously modelled, or topics that are motivating for the learner.

Communicative Competencies

Janice Light (1989) identified key competencies required for learners using aided language to effectively use their AAC systems. These need to be considered when thinking how to teach symbolic language for your learners. Communicative competency is defined as 'the state of being functionally adequate in daily communication and of having sufficient knowledge, judgment, and skills to communicate effectively in daily life' (Light, 1989). This can be split into four main areas: Linguistic, Operational, Social and Strategic competency.

This table has been adapted from Kovach, 2009.

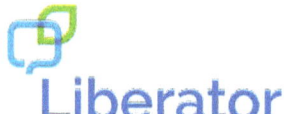

You

Use in language

A frequently occurring core word across all age groups, "you" can be an incredibly effective word to refer to people whose names may not have been programmed onto a device – or indeed people whose names we may not know!

Let's look at some examples in everyday speech:

- Hey **you**!
- I see **you**
- **You** go
- **You** look good

Teaching the word

As a single word "you" can be great to indicate turns and possession. It can be paired well with "me" to demonstrate contrast.

Pronouns can be tricky and it can help when modelling "you" to point to yourself to the other person to emphasise meaning of the word.

Play a sorting game with the PWU AAC. Take a pack of matching pairs cards and create a 'bingo' board for each of you using one set of the matching pairs, putting the other set in a bag. Choose a card from the bag and ask, "Who has this picture?". Encourage the PWU AAC to say, "you" to indicate if you have the matching card which can be paired – the first to pair all their cards wins!

When taking turns in group activities model "you" in response to asking, "Who's turn?", encouraging the PWU AAC to use "you" to indicate whose turn it is. In fun activities let the PWU AAC choose who gets to have a turn by saying "you" and gesturing to the person in question.

Look at personal photographs or videos and ask, "who's that?" encouraging the PWU AAC to respond with "you" when they see you.

> Modelling and aided input is an important part of intervention. When asking questions, modelling the desired response or giving your own response try use the AAC device in addition to your own speech.
>
> Remember that when teaching new vocabulary there needs to be a combination of modelling and allowing the person you support to use the vocabulary. Swap roles – let the person you support both be directed and be the director!

Figure 8.5 This image shows a page from Liberator with the title.

Source: Image courtesy of Liberator Ltd. All rights reserved.

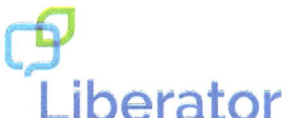

Colouring

Equipment
- Colouring pens or crayons
- Colouring books / plain paper

Vocabulary

Core – I, you, want, that, help, more, again, don't, stop, go, like, make, it, look, wow!

Fringe – (colours)

What to do

Choose a picture from the colouring book you want to colour in. Either do a picture together or choose one each.

Sabotage the pencils crayons by blunting some nibs. Choose pens with tight fitting tops that the PWU AAC will need help opening.

Make silly shapes with your crayons. Do pencil races and 'race' around the paper making the pencil 'stop' and 'go'.

Talk about where different colours are going to go in the picture.

Sentence Ideas
1WL – want, that, help, go, stop, like, (colours)
2WL – want that, want help, like that, make go, like it, look that, want (colours),
3WL – I like it, I want that, I want help, make it go, want it again, I want (colours)

Language Functions
Requesting – want, want (colour), I want (colour)
Directing – go, make go, make it go
Commenting – like, like (colour), I like (colour)
Questioning – like? like (colour)? you like colour?)
Interjecting - wow!

Generalisation
Extend the colours vocabulary into other areas when there are choices or different colours you can see.
Use similar target sentences during art and craft activities.
Play with pavement chalks outside and draw patterns on the path.

Figure 8.6 This image shows a page from Liberator with the heading colouring.

Source: Image courtesy of Liberator Ltd. All rights reserved.

Operational competence	Linguistic competence
- Technical skills used to operate the communication system - Access to the system (e.g. direct selection, scanning) - Use of the communication system functions (e.g. on/off, volume, clear etc.) - Skills to use the system most efficiently	- Learning the language of the home and community (expressive and receptive) - Learning symbols that represent vocabulary and the way vocabulary is organised in the communication system - Combining words into sentences - Range of language functions (e.g. requesting, commenting, greeting, protesting and sharing information)
Social competence - Participating in conversation - Discourse strategies (e.g. initiating, turn-taking) - Expressing different interaction functions (e.g., expressing wants and needs, sharing information, expressing emotions, commenting, protesting etc.)	**Strategic competence** - Using the most appropriate communication method and vocabulary for the situation - Developing compensatory strategies for effective communication with the communication system and any restriction to a learner using the communication system - Repairing communication breakdown

Three main elements support a learner in achieving these competencies. You cannot expect the learner to achieve these alone. To enable these elements to be successfully met, there needs to be the right mix of support from communication partners, the learner themselves and their AAC system. This is shown in the following image. If one of the legs of the stool were to break, or wasn't there, then the whole stool would fall.

It can be tempting to focus on closed questioning when supporting an AAC user linked to the curriculum, rather than a communication focus. It is important to note that it is essential to employ the learners AAC device to use open-ended questioning and building their communication skills, rather than the situation becoming a matter of right or wrong answers. If the AAC user is employing their system solely for an educational activity, they are then unable to communicate. What if they want to comment on what they are doing? Want to express how they're feeling, or what they want or need? This does not allow the learner to communicate with a full range of language functions.

The ultimate aim for an AAC user is to be able to initiate and maintain conversations using a wealth of vocabulary and language functions to enable the user to convey their thoughts and feelings. This is often referred to as 'SNUG' Spontaneous Novel Utterance Generation. At this stage the AAC user has full autonomy over their communication, being able to create unique messages relevant to the given context. This is where true independence in communication is achieved. At this stage communication becomes a natural process of sharing autonomous thought between the AAC user and communication partners.

Conclusion

This chapter considered different strategies that can be used to teach symbolic language. This included the importance of assigning meaning to individual symbols, using the strategy of modelling to support this. There are several resources you can explore to build your confidence when modelling using aided language, which are included in this chapter. The use of modelling aided language for language development will be continued in the next chapter.

Bibliography

Assistiveware (2023). *Core word teaching strategies.* Available at: www.assistiveware.com/learn-aac/learn-about-core-word-teaching-strategies (Accessed: 14 January 2024).

Farrall, J. (2014). *AAC: Systemic change for individual success.* Available at: www.janefarrall.com/aac-systemic-change-for-individual-success/ (Accessed: 14 January 2024).

Kovach, T. (2009). *AAC profile: A continuum of learning.* Pro-ED.

Liberator (no date). *Teaching core words across the day.* Available format: https://liberator.co.uk/media/pdf/TeachingCoreWordsAcrosstheDay-2019.pdf (Accessed: January 2024).

Light, J. (1989). Toward a Definition of Communicative Competence for Individuals Using Augmentative and Alternative Communication Systems. *Augmentative and Alternative Communication*, 5(2), pp.137–144.

Porter, G. (2004). Chatting at school? Proceedings-ISAAC conference, Natal Brazil.

9 Modelling

Lack of staff is a marked hurdle when supporting those with complex Speech, Language and Communication Needs (SLCN) using Augmentative and Alternative Communication (AAC) as has been identified throughout this book. Teachers can often find it challenging to know how to support these learners and effectively model using their AAC systems without the guidance of a Speech and Language Therapist. This is particularly true for early career teachers, or those who have had no prior experience of aided language/AAC within their classroom. Teachers can feel overwhelmed by the prospect of needing to meet the needs of the learner, whilst also meeting the needs of their peers.

In this chapter we will consider what modelling is and how to use this in your classroom to best support your learners.

What is Modelling?

The strategy of modelling often has different labels, for example, aided language simulation, aided language input and point talking. In this book the term modelling will be used to encompass all these approaches.

For many years modelling has been identified consistently within research as a technique for teaching language and increasing the responsiveness and use of aided language/AAC for learners with Speech, Language and Communication Needs (Binger and Light, 2007; Beck et al., 2009). Learners who use aided language/AAC are shown to make rapid gains in their aided language production when they are exposed to modelling (Binger et al., 2008, pg. 110). This can be due to "A child who uses AAC will independently select the words she wishes to use from the vocabulary other people have chosen to model and, for aided symbols, made available for her to use" (Porter and Kirkland, 1995).

Modelling generally involves the use of the child's AAC system, although in some circumstances different symbol communication boards may be used by the communication partner – for example a core board or activity-specific aided language displays. Examples of this could include a communication board relating to a game or the topic being studied.

Modelling can involve the following:

- The use of symbols to say real things in real situations
- What to say and when to say it
- The use of grammar
- How to use the device
- Mistakes and repair strategies

Beginning Modelling

When first beginning to model it can seem like an overwhelming prospect, but remember you are not alone! We have all been there at some point and continue to learn and make mistakes along the way! Don't put too much pressure on yourself to get it right from the start and model everything you say. To support you in the early days, make sure you are prepared. If the learner is new to your class or has just been given a new AAC system, it can be challenging to know where to find vocabulary within the system, how to navigate to the correct page, even with the handy tool, 'find word', feature seen on most electronic communication aids. Make sure you have spent time getting to know the system and have an idea of where to find vocabulary you wish to model. If the child will not let you hold their electronic AAC communication aid, many suppliers have software which can be used on a computer to simulate the vocabulary and make edits. This will give you the opportunity to explore the vocabulary when the learner is also not present, for example once they have gone home. Many suppliers have created paper-based versions of their vocabularies to be used alongside the learner's electronic AAC. Some of these are more detailed than others, but just by having access to the paper-based version of the vocabularies' top page (often their 'core page') there is so much rich language you can model, particularly core vocabulary which can be used in any given situation and is non-context specific. Be persistent and don't give up hope! Over time 'practice makes perfect!'

> **Discussion Point!**
>
> Think about a learner you are supporting to use aided language/AAC within a particular lesson or activity. Looking at some of the core word information in the earlier chapters, which core words would be most relevant to model? Ensure you are modelling a range of language functions.

Using the AAC system alongside the spoken word may not come naturally at first, but remember you don't need to model every single word, and it does not need to be grammatically correct – just some key words within each sentence. For example, when saying, 'It's time for dinner!', simply point to 'time' and 'dinner', or just 'dinner' as this is the key bit of information in the sentence. Everyone is learning together, including the learner themselves, so it is important to be open and honest about this and show that you are not an expert on the vocabulary. This will lower the user's anxieties that they have to get everything right. Talk out loud your thoughts as to where to find vocabulary, for example for 'dinner' you may say:

'Hmmm … I'm not sure where to find dinner on the device, let's take a look. Let's look in topics. I can see one called "food". I think dinner may be in here as you eat food for dinner. Let's see if it's in there. I can see lots of different foods in here. If I look at the top I can see breakfast, snacks, meals, puddings. Ah! There's dinner!'

If you get stuck, that's okay, and it is important you show the learner this. But also, to show how this can be fixed, for example:

'Oops! That's the wrong page! It's okay, I can go back into topics and take another look. I'm not sure where to find dinner, let's look. Ahh! There it is!'

By verbalising your thoughts in this way, you are teaching the learner it's okay to make mistakes, but also operational skills to support them in navigating around the vocabulary independently. This will enable them to feel more confident to explore the vocabulary to find chosen words, rather than passively waiting for the communication partner to show them where to find them. Although prompting was discussed in the previous chapter, it is worth noting that when considering how to approach modelling with a learner, ensure you're providing them with the least amount of prompting necessary for the task. If you over-prompt then this can cause the learner to become reliant on this, rather than working towards using the AAC system independently to initiate autonomous communication.

When teaching specific curriculum vocabulary, rather than focussing on specific topic words, such as *volcano*, use vocabulary on the device which can be used in varying contexts; for example, instead navigate towards 'hot' and 'hill' to describe the volcano. In future, the learner will then remember the pathway for 'hot' and use this in different ways, for example to describe if the weather is hot, they're feeling hot, or the food is hot. By doing so, you do not have to continually update the AAC system with topic-based vocabulary which may be used only on a few occasions, saving you time! This also means the learner has learnt how to locate vocabulary they will need to use on a regular basis.

Descriptive Teaching

This approach is often referred to as the 'Descriptive Teaching Model' (Van Tatenhove, 2008). Using a descriptive style, the teacher mentions and references the context-specific words, then teaches concepts behind the words using high-frequency, re-usable common words. In this case the learner describes the word, focussing on the concept. This is in contrast to teaching.

Referential style	Descriptive style
Requires large vocabulary of words rarely needed in daily life	Focusses on a smaller vocabulary which is used in daily life
Rote learning requires the least amount of effort	Requires creative thinking about how to describe the concept with available vocabulary
High memory demand, but with little payoff and generalisation into real life situations	Focusses on the information shared in the lesson rather than on new pages and symbols within the learner's AAC system

Discussion Point!

Looking at these concepts relating to the Ancient Egyptians. Which of these frequency words would you use to describe the words listed?

Concept	Descriptive method
Hieroglyphics	
Tutankhamun	
Pharaoh	
Mummification	
Canopic jars	
Sphinx	

Types of Modelling

There are three main types of modelling to use: personal modelling, modelling to attribute meaning, and modelling to extend a communication attempt.

Personal Modelling

- This can be used each time you interact with the learner and use their AAC system in naturally occurring situations throughout the learner's day.
- There is no expectation to model every word and navigate to this on the learner's AAC system. Instead, model a few words, preferably from the core vocabulary.

Imagine you are delivering an art lesson, using the Project Core board shown in Figure 9.1: Try to make a few phrases you could model whilst you are teaching the learners:
How many phrases did you come up with? Here are some examples:

- Do you **want** me to **help** you **open** the paint?
- Do you **want** some **more** paint?
- **Look** at your picture!
- **I like** your picture!

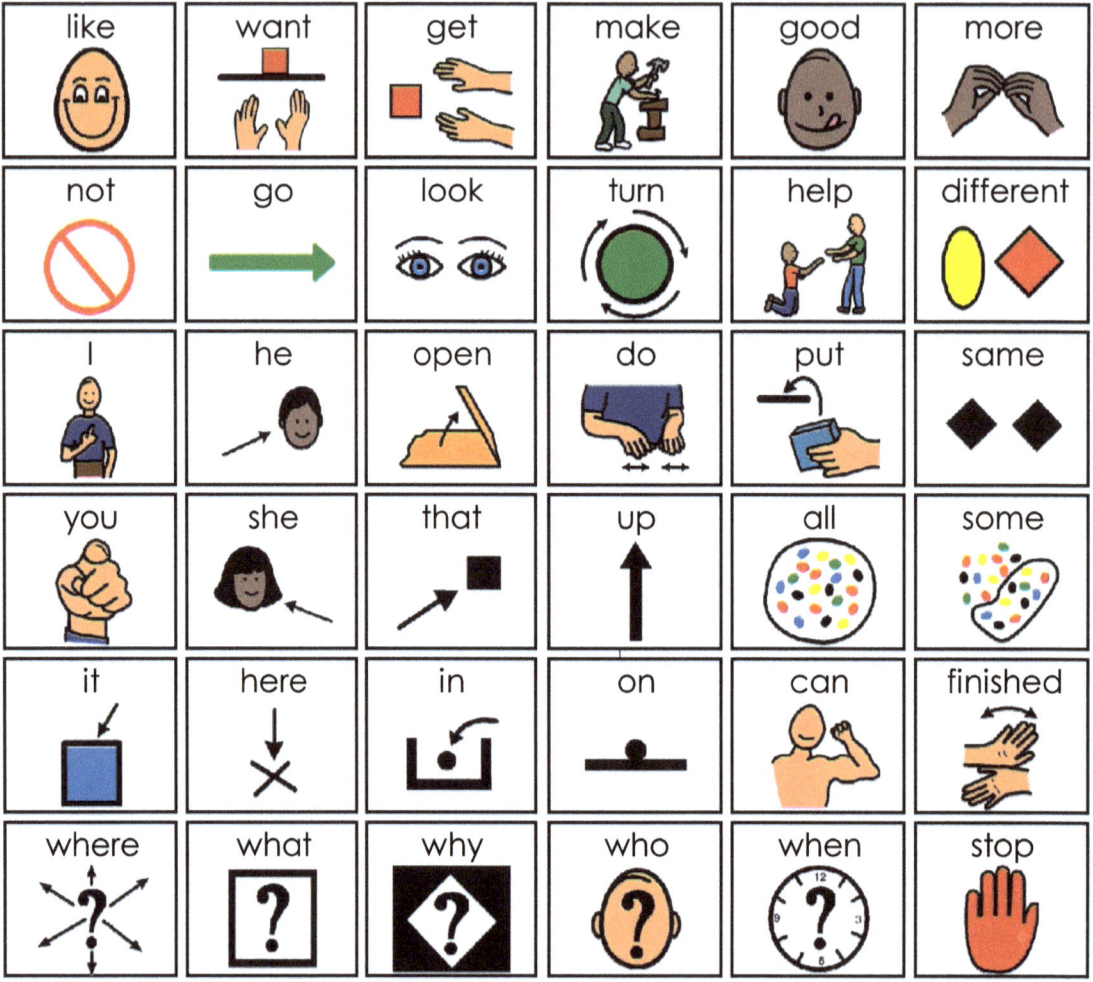

Figure 9.1 Image of 36 symbols on a white background.

Source: University of North Carolina at Chapel Hill, The Center for Literacy and Disability Studies. www.project-core.com

- Can you **put** the paint **here?**
- It's time to **finish** painting.

Modelling to Attribute Meaning

- This is often used for early communicators and for those with complex communication needs, who are not yet able to use a robust AAC system.
- This form of modelling picks up on a learner's non-verbal communication – for example, their vocalisations and changes in their pitch and volume, gesturing towards an item or leading an adult towards something.
- The role of the communication partner is to identify what the learner may be trying to communicate through their actions and assign meaning to this onto their AAC system, modelling where to find relevant vocabulary. This requires the communication partner to make good use of their observation skills.

For example:

- Learner: *Crying*
- Communication partner: *You look **sad.***

- Learner: *Hand leading towards the books*
- Communication partner: *You look like you want to **read** a book.*

- Learner: *Running towards the door*
- Communication partner: *You look like you **want** to **go** outside.*

- Learner: *Pushing away a toy*
- Communication partner: *You look like you **want** to **finish.***

- Learner: *Scrunching up face when trying a food*
- Communication partner: *You look like you **don't like** that!*

- Learner: *Laughing during an activity*
- Communication partner: *You look like you **like** that!*

- Learner: *Reaching for more bricks when building a tower*
- Communication partner: *You look like you **want more** bricks.*

> **Discussion Point!**
>
> Consider the learners in your classroom, who are using mainly their body language to communicate.
>
> - What do you think they may be communicating?
> - Can you assign meaning by using aided language?
> - Have you put something in place for these learners to aid their communication?
> - If they have not been understood, how do they react?

Scaffolding: Modelling to Extend a Communication Attempt

- This is appropriate for learners who already have an AAC system in place, whether this be paper-based or electronic.
- The communication partner needs to model one symbol above what they are communicating. For example, if they are using just one symbol, combine two together, or if they are using two, model using three symbols. This keeps you ahead of the game and continues to push language development.

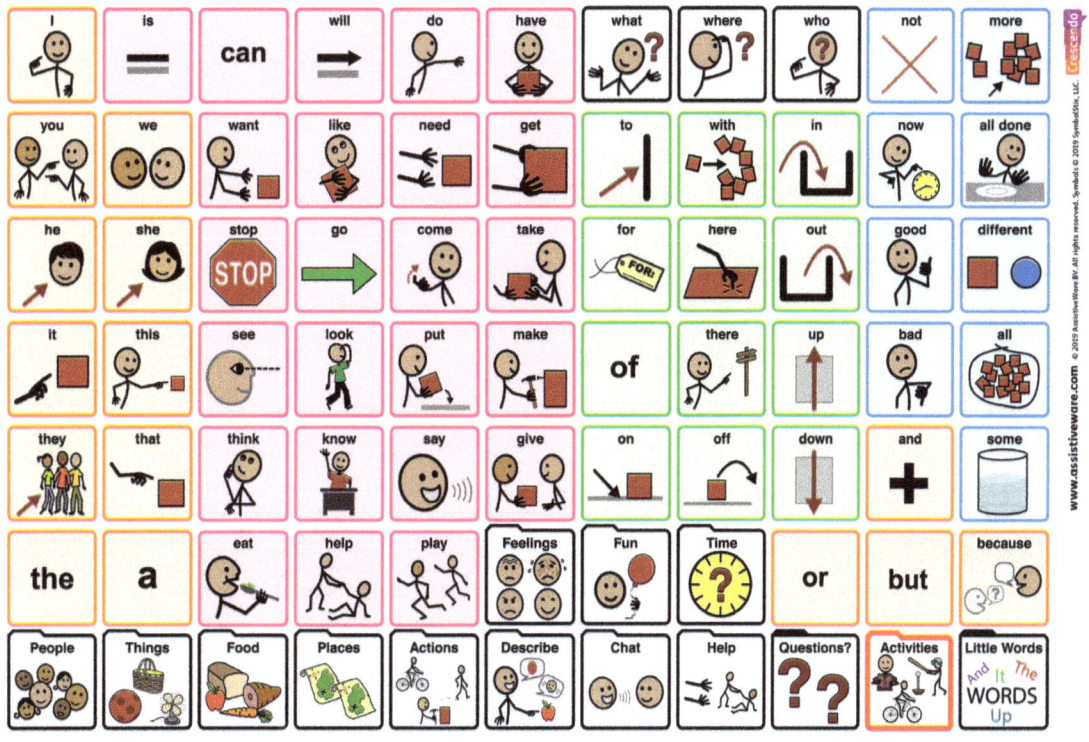

Figure 9.2 This image shows a communication chart with 77 symbols.

Source: www.assistiveware.com ©2019 AssistiveWare BV. All rights reserved. Symbols © 2019 SymbolStix, LLC.

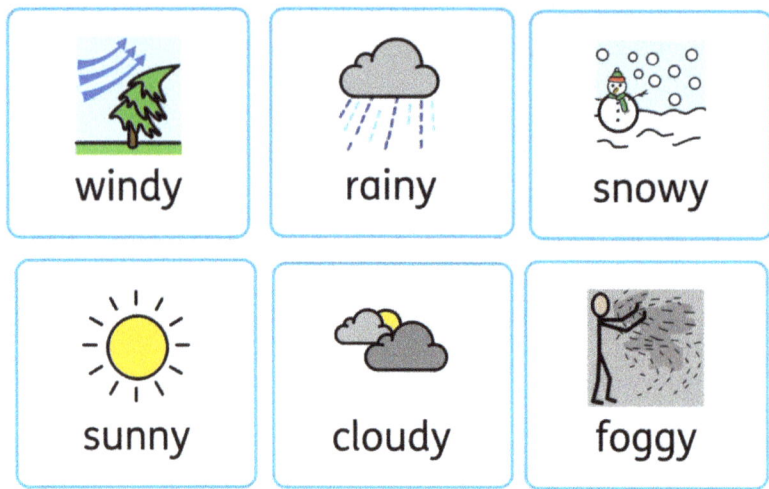

Figure 9.3 This image shows 6 weather symbols.

Source: Widgit Symbols © Widgit Software Ltd 2002–2023. www.widgit.com

For example, consider a circle time session talking about the weather. You have the symbols for windy, rainy, snowy, sunny, cloudy and foggy on the board (Figure 9.2). Rather than the learner choosing just the correct symbol for the weather outside, focus on combining symbols together. Figure 9.3 is an example of the core board within the ProloQuo2Go vocabulary, which can be used as a stand-alone, paper-based printout, or an app on an iPad, which can be used electronically.

For example:

- Learner: *Sunny*
- Communication partner: *I can **see** that it is **sunny** today.*

- Learner: *Rainy*
- Communication partner: *I want it to **stop** being **rainy** today!*

- Learner: *Where sun?*
- Communication partner: ***Where** did the **sun go**?*

- Learner: *Play snowy*
- Communication partner: *Do you **want** to **play** in the **snow**?*

- Learner: *Want stop rainy*
- Communication partner: *Do you **want** it to **stop raining here**?*

- Learner: *Not see fog*
- Communication partner: ***You** can **not see when** it is foggy*

Modelling AAC versus Forcing the use of AAC

The differences between these can be seen below.

Modelling AAC	Forcing AAC
Model what the learner could say.	Insisting on the use of the learner's AAC system. The communication partner halts the interaction until the learner has complied, e.g asking a learner whether they want a banana or an apple and withholding the food items until they have used their AAC system to identify which they would like.
Take time and make use of pauses to give the learner the opportunity to respond, without expecting or demanding it.	Forcing the learner to use their AAC system using hand over hand, removing their autonomy e.g. during the lesson identifying shapes, using hand over hand to force the learner to point to 'circle' when showing them the circle.

Modelling AAC	Forcing AAC
Allow opportunities for the learner to participate.	Giving up too early without allowing time for the learner to develop the skills required to use their AAC system, e.g., after just a few sessions or weeks, as the learner has not responded using their AAC system, coming to the conclusion that the AAC system is too complex for them and they do not have the skills to access it. Learning language takes time.
Use repetition, across contexts; for example, talk about feeling hot, the hot weather, hot food. Facilitate this in different environments and with a variety of communication partners.	Forcing the learner to respond, despite having modelled the response to the learner, e.g. expecting the learner to express their emotions using their AAC system during a circle time session, without having previously modelled with the learner and shown the pathway to navigate to appropriate vocabulary and assigning meaning to the individual symbols.
Model the use of core vocabulary rather than focussing on nouns; use descriptive teaching rather than focusing on topic vocabulary.	Insisting the learner create full and grammatically correct sentences which take a long time to construct and can stop the flow of interaction. For example, 'I **went** to the supermarket', using **went** rather than 'go'.
Use a total communication approach, accepting all forms of communication, for example speech, vocalisations, signing, body language, use of AAC system	Forcing the learner to use their communication, even when they have expressed what they wish to say verbally/through their body language and you have understood what they are saying; e.g. if the learner has gestured that they need the toilet and you understand this, forcing them to find it on their AAC system, which can then lead to them urinating or soiling themselves as you have not responded promptly enough!

Tips for Modelling

When first started out modelling, it could be overwhelming to know the best way of doing so to support your learners. Here's some helpful tips to get you started:

- Start small, don't become bogged down with modelling every word in a sentence. Try modelling a word above what the learner is currently using, for example, if the learner is just saying 'go' extend this to I 'want' to 'go'.
- Don't worry about the grammar when first starting out; begin by using core words which can be used in different contexts.
- Don't just ask questions; ensure you are modelling a range of language functions for example, not just requesting, but instead giving opportunities for commenting, negating, telling stories and so forth.
- Don't put pressure on yourself to model all day.
- Make sure you are modelling on the learner's AAC system (or a copy of this, whether electronic or paper-based).
- Ensure that their AAC system is always available – it is not out of reach or in a cupboard! If it is an electronic communication aid, ensure that it is also turned on and charged, ready to use!
- Don't worry if the learner isn't looking. They may be using their peripheral vision or taking in the auditory feedback. You are modelling not only where to access vocabulary on the device and navigate to the correct word, but also the language itself.
- Don't become perturbed; it can take time for a learner to use their device and that is okay!

If you have just one learner in your classroom who uses AAC, it can be challenging to model for them to use their system whilst also supporting all learners in your classroom. It can be helpful engaging in group modelling. This gives the clear message to learners and staff, that using aided language/AAC is a worthwhile and valued as a form of communication. Using modelling with all learners, not just those with an AAC system can support teaching and learning for all learners.

Imagine a lesson you are teaching to the whole class, for example outer space. Figure 9.4 is a screenshot of the space page within the WordPower vocabulary used on Liberator devices, for example, NovaChats, as well as through TouchChat on the iPad.

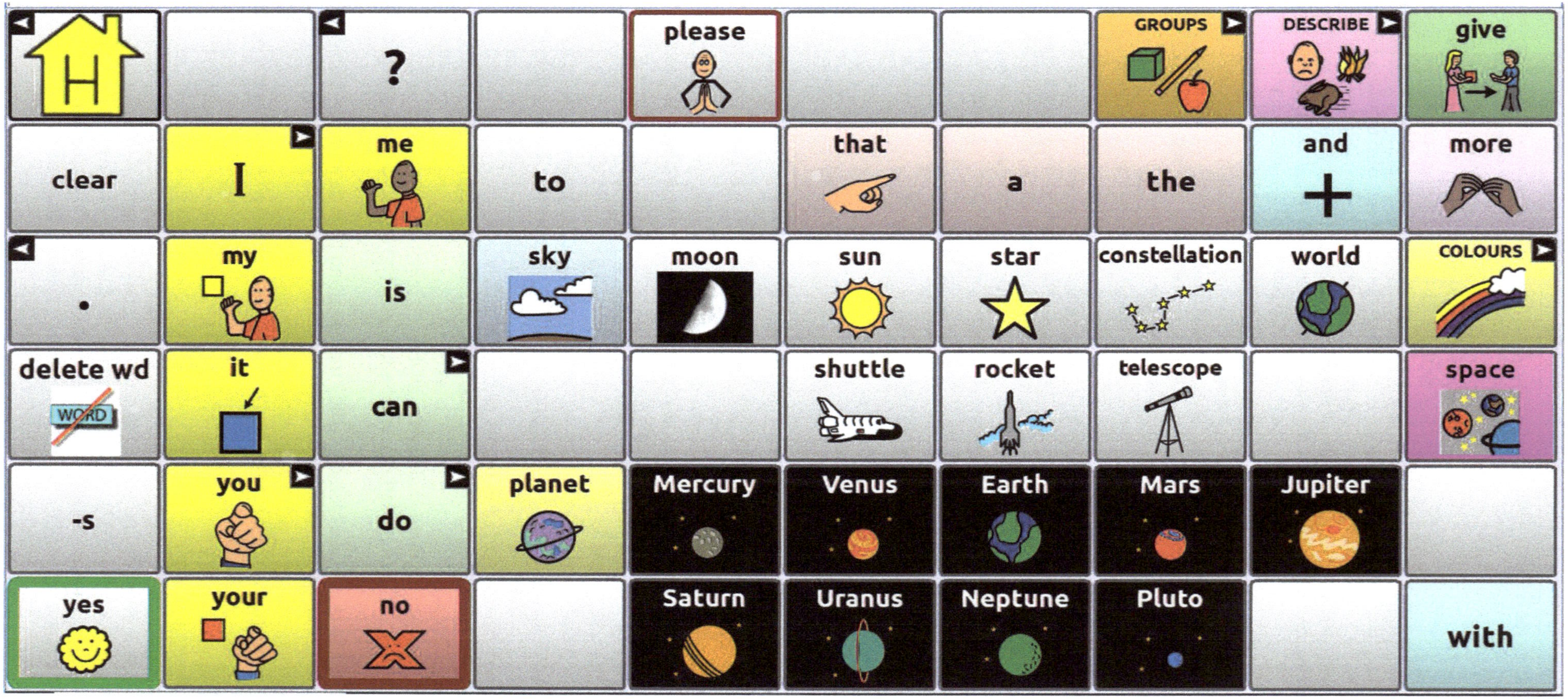

Figure 9.4 This image shows a screenshot of a vocabulary with words related to space.

Source: Image courtesy of Liberator Ltd. All rights reserved. Symbols included are SymbolStix ® Copyright © 2023 SymbolStix, LLC. All rights reserved. Used with Permission.

Consider when supporting the whole class that the page can support not only the learner who uses the communication aid but can also support their peers in the generation of ideas. The symbols offer a visual prompt for learners to support the generation of ideas, rather than having to think of ideas from scratch, retrieving the information required independently. This provides the vocabulary that is relevant to the topic.

Assistiveware have created a great poster sharing the 'Do's and Don'ts for AAC', (Figure 9.5) which can be displayed in your classroom as a reminder (Enders, 2013). Enders also created the 'AAC Bootcamp' resource, available here https://aaccommunity.net/2017/08/aac-boot-camp/, which is also a good reminder of strategies to use which can be displayed in the classroom. These are particularly helpful as a reminder of what to do when modelling, but also for unfamiliar communication partners – for example, new staff or supply staff in your classroom. Teamwork can make all the difference when modelling, ensuring everyone is on the same page and working together, and consistently, to support the learner. Points to consider include:

- Ensuring you are creating a positive environment, where learners' AAC systems are valued and respected, having a positive attitude towards aided language and the learner's AAC system.
- Model using the AAC system yourself so that staff can see its importance and will be more willing to give it a go as they have seen examples of modelling within the classroom.
- Ensure you are providing staff with adequate information and training to ensure they are confident in supporting the learner.
- Embed modelling into everyday classroom practice, rather than its being seen as an add-on and something additional to implement in the classroom.
- Appreciate that the learner is acquiring a new skill, and this can be difficult at times, but is something that will improve with modelling in place. Compliment staff when you see good practice in order to grow their confidence.
- Set the expectation that staff will model. Remind them of the importance of this throughout the day; for example, 'Did you get an opportunity to use Katy's AAC system when you went out to the shops? Let's take it to the café tomorrow'.

Modelling versus Structured Lessons

It can feel overwhelming to think about how and when you are going to implement structure sessions to support the learner in developing their skills and use of their AAC system, but modelling does not need to be planned out in advance – put less pressure on yourself as a teacher. Modelling incidentally throughout the day can have a far greater impact on the learner.

Modelling	Structured sessions
This mimics more natural conversation and typical language development. It allows for the development of social communication e.g. chatting with friends.	This focusses on specific vocabulary, which is often topic-based (rather than a high-frequency vocabulary) and can be generalised and used in any context or conversation.
There is less pressure on both the communication partner and the learner themselves to get it right as this occurs incidentally rather than having a key focus.	Adds pressure on the communication partner and learner as there is a focus on teaching specific vocabulary, and can turn the learning task and acquisition of vocabulary into something which is either right or wrong.
Modelling can be far less time consuming than being required to think of something more specific. Modelling can occur across the day, not just within lessons, so there is no need to timetable this as additional time in the day.	Time consuming as the structured sessions need to be thought through and planned in advance of the session, ensuring any resources which are required have been created before the session and are ready to use.
As modelling occurs naturally, there is no time needed in order to focus on creating relevant resources. Specific communication lessons do not need to be planned into the day.	

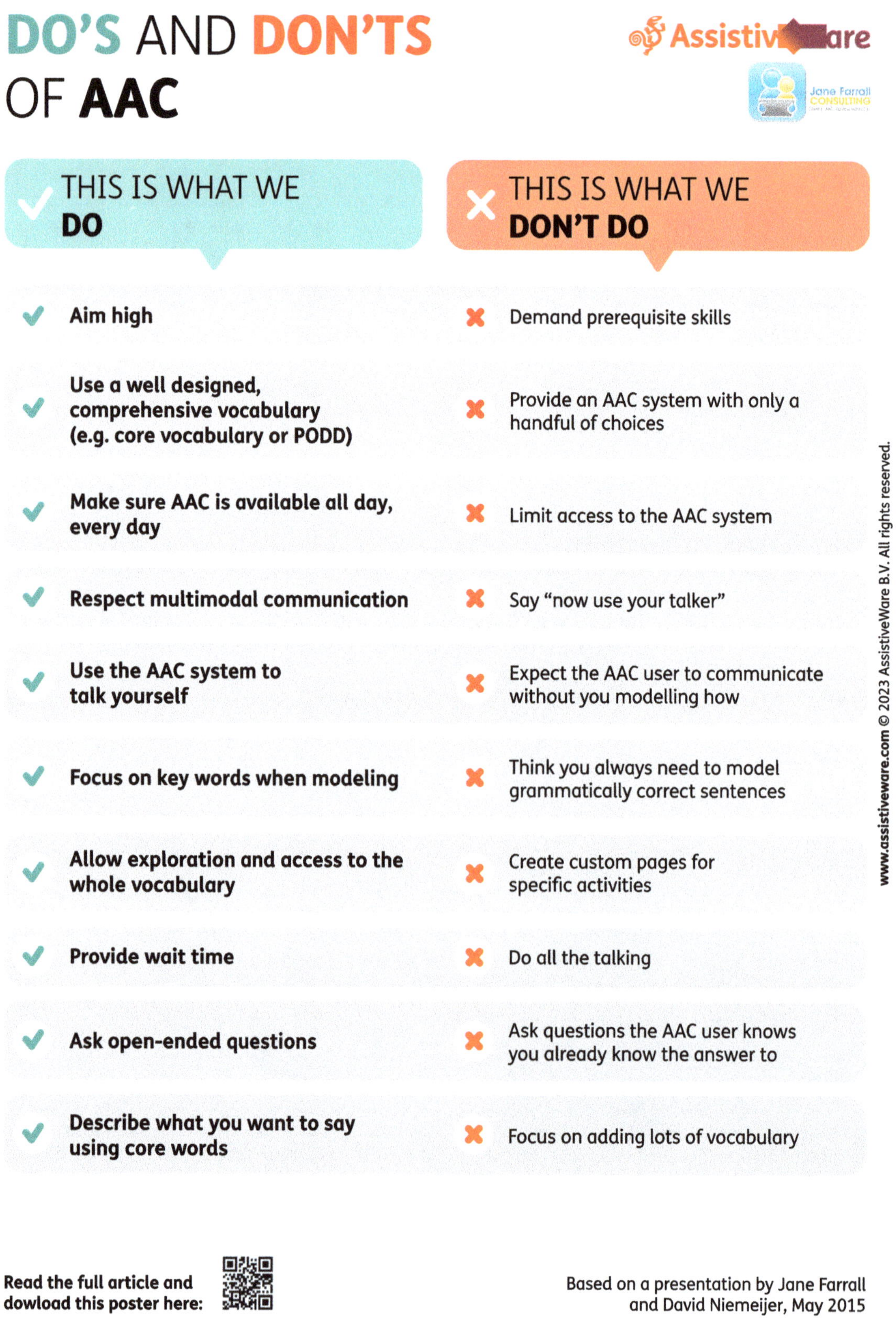

Figure 9.5 This image shows the Dos and Don'ts of AAC.

Source: www.assistiveware.com ©2023 AssistiveWare B.V. All rights reserved.

Peer Modelling

In addition to communication partners modelling for learners, there is huge power in peer modelling. Peers can be taught to be successful communication partners from a young age. This provides learners with increased opportunities to develop their social communication, benefiting both the peer and learner with an AAC system to become more competent in their social interactions (Bourque, 2020). Integrating peer modelling will help the learner to learn a larger repertoire of not just vocabulary, but also communicative functions (Bourque and Goldstein, 2020).

Learners can build connections between symbols on their AAC systems and spoken words, assigning meaning to what they represent when peers use the learner's AAC system alongside them (Drager, 2009; Wood et al., 1998).

To support peer modelling:

- Provide frequent opportunities for the learners to communicate with each other socially, for example chatting and gossiping! This will ensure communication is functional for the learner.
- Create activities which promote communication between the learners.

Case Study

Megan and Louise (Figures 9.6.and 9.7) both use the EasyChat60 vocabulary on an Accent 800. Louise has the symbol stix symbol set, whereas Megan uses the Widgit symbols and also uses a touch guide to support her access.

Louise had been using EasyChat for several years before Megan received her device. Megan would not let adults near her device. She would often say 'mine' and cuddle her device. Staff working alongside her were creative when it came to modelling, for example using paper-based resources to model with her. Although she wouldn't let adults near her device, she was happy for Louise to do so as her peer. As Louise had been using the

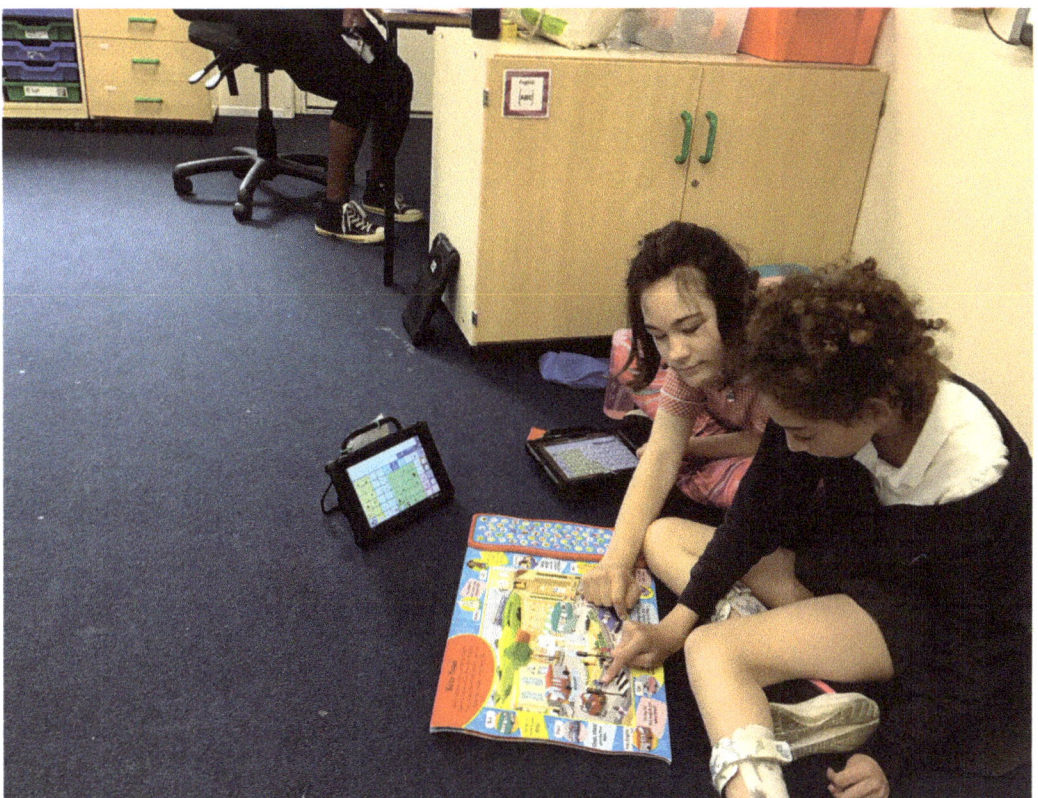

Figure 9.6 This image shows 2 girls with their communication aids.

Source: Photographed by the author.

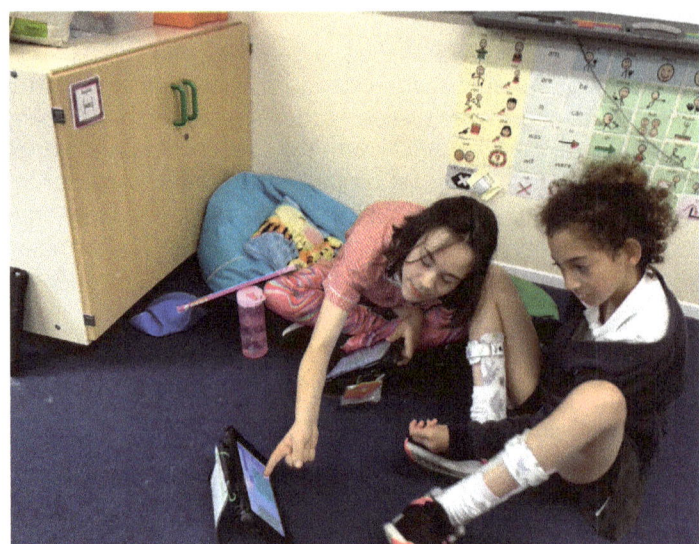

Figure 9.7 This image shows 2 girls with their communication aids.

Source: Photographed by the author.

vocabulary for sometime she was confident in showing Megan where to locate vocabulary. Due to this, Megan became efficient and used the device functionally within social communication. Louise and Megan would have girly chats and even argue using their devices away from adults. They would share books together and discuss them as a pair independently. In time, not only did Louise show Megan where to locate vocabulary, but as Megan became more familiar she also showed Louise where relevant vocabulary was. Both learners grew in confidence as they were learning from each other rather than in structured sessions with an adult. They were able to interact socially not just with each other and with other peers in the classroom, but with those in different classes. Megan particularly enjoyed interacting with older verbal pupils. They again were able to model on Megan's device and expand her social communication.

Conclusion

Learners benefit significantly from the use of modelling to support their use of aided language and it promotes language development. This can be carried out by both adults and peers in different contexts. Modelling doesn't need to be an additional task through structured communication lessons. Naturally occurring interactions are far more powerful in developing the learner's confidence when using their AAC system and locating relevant vocabulary. In the moment, modelling allows communication partners to attribute meaning to the aided language in a way that is not onerous for the learner or communication partner.

Next, we are going to do a deeper dive into the different functions of language, considering the reasons why we communication and how to avoid the pitfall of focussing heavily on requesting an object, for example, during snack time, requesting food items – 'I want biscuit'.

Bibliography

Beck, A., Stoner, J. and Dennis, M. (2009). An Investigation of Aided Language Stimulation: Does it Increase AAC Use with Adults with Developmental Disabilities and Complex Communication Needs? *Augmentative and Alternative Communication*, 25(1), pp.42–54.

Binger, C. and Light, J. (2007). The Effect of Aided AAC Modeling on the Expression of Multi-Symbol Messages by Preschoolers Who Use AAC. *Augmentative and Alternative Communication*, 23(1), pp.30–43.

Binger, C., Berens, J., Kent-Walsh, J. and Taylor, S. (2008). The Effects of Aided AAC Interventions on AAC Use, Speech and Symbolic Gestures. *Seminars in Speech and Language*, 29(2), pp.101–111.

Bourque, K. (2020). Peer-Mediated Augmentative and Alternative Communication Interventions for Young Children With Autism Spectrum Disorder and Limited to No Spoken Communication. *Perspectives of the ASHA Special Interest Groups*, 5(3), pp.602–610.

Bourque, K. and Goldstein, H. (2020). Expanding Communication Modalities and Functions for Preschoolers With Autism Spectrum Disorder: Secondary Analysis of a Peer Partner Speech-Generating Device Intervention. *Journal of Speech Language and Hearing Research*, 63(3), pp.1–16.

Drager, K. (2009). Aided Modeling Interventions for Children With Autism Spectrum Disorders Who Require AAC. *Perspectives on Augmentative and Alternative Communication*, 18(4), pp.114.

Enders, L. (2013). *AAC Bootcamp*. Available at: https://talklink.org.nz/uploads/08f9785abd39cda87ed8529803ed1de3.pdf (Accessed 14 January 2024).

Porter, G. and Kirkland, J. (1995). *Integrating augmentative and alternative communication into group programs: Utilizing the principles of conductive Education*. Melbourne: Spastic Society of Victoria.

Van Tatenhove, G.M. and Arrington, B. (2008). *Aided language stimulation and the descriptive teaching model*. Montreal: ISAAC.

Wood, L., Lasker, J., Siegel-Causey, E., Beukelman, D. and Ball, L. (1998). An Input Framework For Augmentative and Alternative Communication. *Augmentative and Alternative Communication*, 14, pp.261–267.

10 Language Development: The Danger Zone of Just Requesting

This chapter focuses specifically on learners who need support with language development. Some of your learners will be typical with their language development, in that they would communicate for a wide range of purposes, if they were able to use verbal speech. Teaching your learner aided language and giving them access to this to express themselves will allow you to clearly see who needs additional support with language development.

The most important thing to remember when we are thinking about language development with using aided language is that we want the person to be able to achieve autonomous communication. If you remember back to earlier in this book, we can say that autonomous communication is when the young person can communicate anything they want to say to whoever they want to say it to, whenever they want to say it (Porter, 2018).

An aided language user may need to develop their language skills because they are still young and at the early stages of their language development journey. Alternatively, it could be because they have a language delay.

This chapter will do a deeper dive into how you can support language development in the classroom.

The learner's speech and language therapist should work alongside you in a multidisciplinary team to offer personalised guidance and support around profiling and target setting for that learner. However, if you find yourself working without adequate access to speech and language therapy support, this chapter will signpost to some useful profiling tools for thinking about the communicative functions a learner is already using and also how to draw some targets from those profiling tools.

> **Discussion Point!**
>
> Try to imagine coming home after a busy day. Write down or type out some of the things you might say to someone when you are home; this might be your partner, your pet or a friend or relative on the phone.
> - Play out the conversation in your head. What did you talk about? Did you complain? Did you comment on things that happened in the day? Did you ask any questions? Did you request anything? All of these examples link to different functions of language.

We use a range of language functions all the time when we talk. The language function is the reason why we want to communicate. The different functions represent the autonomous thought that we are generating in our heads. What we say to others allows us to express who we are, regulate our emotional state and show others our personality – so it is key to our identity. What we say allows us to function effectively in a range of situations and environments. The different functions of language allow us to communicate with a range of communication partners and helps us to foster relationships with other humans.

Now let's think about aided language you may have seen in classroom environments. The majority will be around receptive language, as discussed in previous chapters, such as visual timetables, now and next boards, social stories, and s forth. You may also have seen choice boards (Figure 10.1), so the learner can express choices in leisure times.

Another popular aided language tool, particularly for a learner with a diagnosis of autism, is PECS – Picture Exchange Communication System (Figure 10.2).

Choice boards and PECS in its earliest stages focus heavily on the language function of requesting. A typical scenario is at break time – a child collects or is given their PECS book or choice board and is asked the closed question: 'What do you want for snack?' The learner will make a selection from the limited choice of symbols made available to them and receive their item of choice. Once finished, everyone tidies up and the PECS book or choice board gets tidied

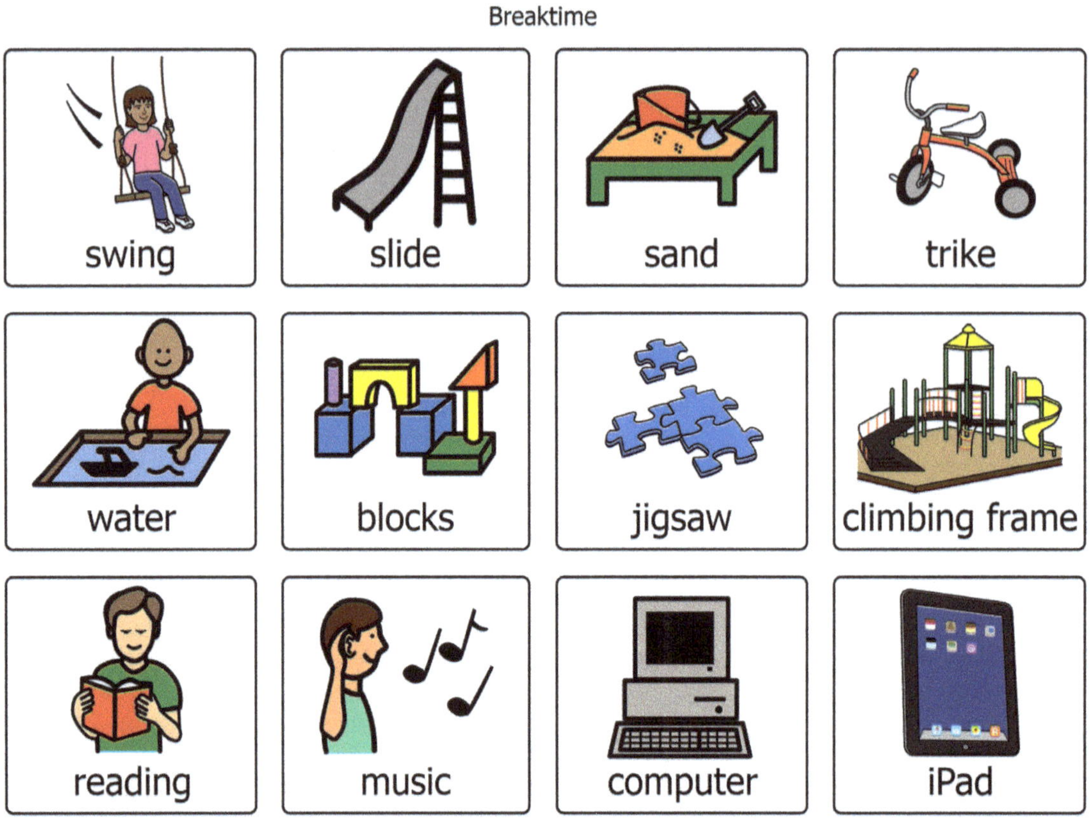

Figure 10.1 A 12 cell choice board labelled 'Breaktime'.

Source: Created by the author using PCS symbols. PCS and Boardmaker are trademarks of Tobii Dynavox LLC. All rights reserved. Used with permission.

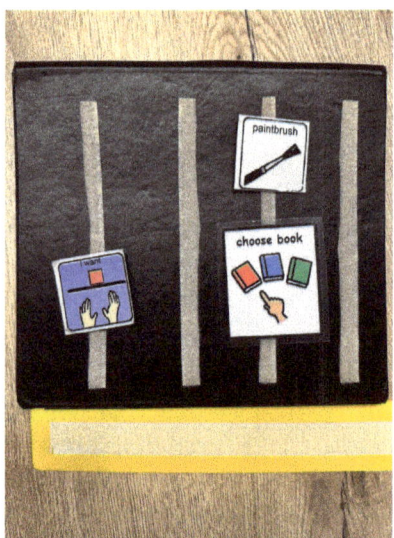

Figure 10.2 A black folder with 3 symbols on the top.

Source: Photographed by the author.

away, too. If the child needed help opening a packet, they would likely reach for a supporting adult and get upset if that gesture was misunderstood. If a child wanted something different, they would probably reach over and take someone else's, upsetting a classmate. If the child did not want any food, they would probably throw the snack on the floor or across the room. By only making accessible aided language to request items, we are not giving the learner the opportunity to use aided language for a range of language functions. Therefore, we are likely to see a suite of behaviours that the child has learnt as effective communication for that language function, for example, 'To reject something, I throw it'.

PECS is often described as a behaviour support rather than a robust communication system. PECS describe themselves as relying "on the principles of applied behaviour analysis (ABA) so that distinct prompting, reinforcement, and error correction strategies are specified at each training phase in order to teach spontaneous, functional communication" (Bondy and Frost, 2001, p. 728). Many autistic adults have spoken up about the harm ABA caused them as children. Shkedy, Shkedy and Sandoval (2021) identified that research shows ABA neglects the structure of the autistic brain, child development, the complexities of human psychology. There has also been a general trend within the fields of education and health to step away from physical touch without informed consent, for example using hand over hand support as is used within the earliest stages of PECS.

A review of evidence for interventions for children on the autism spectrum was commissioned by the National Disability Insurance Agency and completed by Autism CRC, in Australia.

CRC's umbrella review summarised data from systematic reviews of intervention research for children on the autism spectrum, particularly those aged 0–12 years. This showed PECs to offer low quality social communication, expressive language and general outcomes having an overall inconsistent therapeutic effect.

When thinking about aided language tools/Augmentative and Alternative Communication, it is imperative that there is access to symbols that represent all the different functions of language, such as commenting, rejecting and protesting. Otherwise, how can we support the development of that autonomous communication using aided language?

It is worthwhile to draw your attention back to the diagram earlier in the book (Figure 10.3) around the development of pragmatics and think about where your learner with Speech, Language and Communication Needs (SLCN) sits. Do they use all of these communicative functions? Maybe their profile is spikey, and they use some communicative functions but not others.

When thinking about the development of communicative functions, it is worthwhile noting that this is not something often taught to educators. It is only if there has been collaborative teamwork between speech and language therapists and the education team when information around this may have been shared. Otherwise, the class team may feel very much in the dark around language development.

It may be worthwhile to think about having some visual displays in the classroom environment to support understanding around the development of pragmatics (why we communicate) and the different communicative functions. Figure 10.4 is an example of one such visual aid.

Profiling Tools

It is extremely useful for you to have a sound understanding of where your learner currently sits within their language development journey. What communicative functions do they already use? Do they already map verbal, aided or even unaided language onto those communicative functions? For example, a learner may have a unique gesture or sign that they consistently apply meaning to, and which represents a communicative function. A profiling tool can help us to identify what communication a learner is currently offering and how they are currently offering it.

The Pragmatic Profile

> *The Pragmatics Profile of Everyday Communication Skills in Children*, originally developed in 1988 by Hazel Dewart and Susie Summers, has been used extensively by Speech and Language Therapists for many years. It was initially intended for use with pre-school aged children, however it was extended for use with children up to the age of 10 years when a revised edition was published in 1995. *A Pragmatics Profile of Everyday Communication Skills in Adults* was developed in 1996 to provide a way of exploring communication at stages in the lifespan from adolescent to elderly people.
>
> The development of the Profile was intended to provide practitioners with a means of collecting information about a child's communication skills outside the clinical setting, and focused more on their communication abilities in everyday life.
>
> The Profile was based on the pragmatic approach to understanding language which emphasises how communication is achieved, how language is used to communicate a variety of intentions, the related needs of the listener, and how children participate in conversation and discourse.
>
> (Bates 1976, cited in Dewart and Summers 1995)

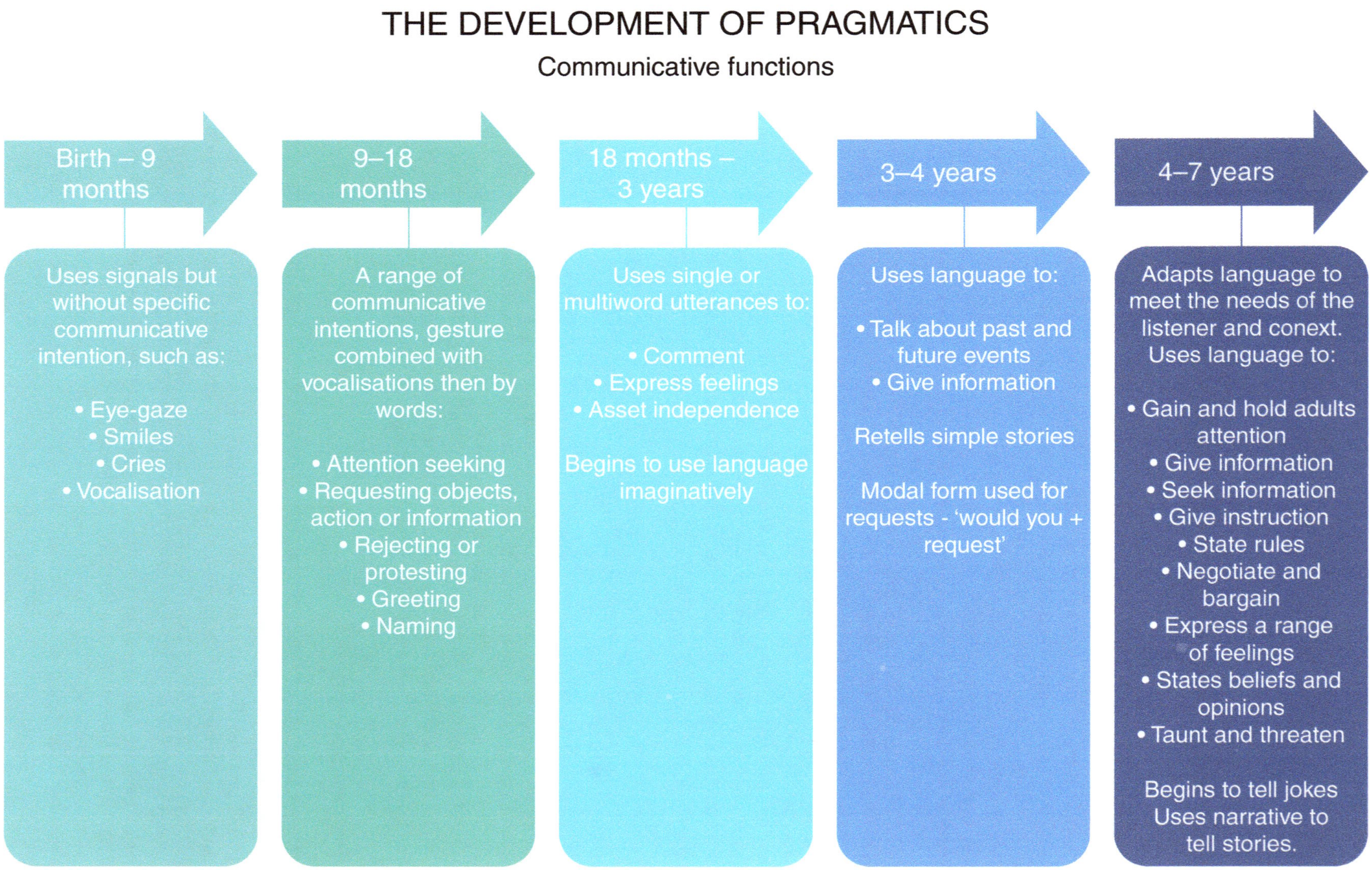

94 *Language Development: The Danger Zone of Just Requesting*

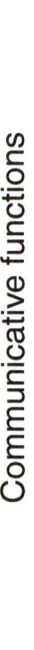

Figure 10.3 An image of 5 developmental stages.

Source: Image created by the author.

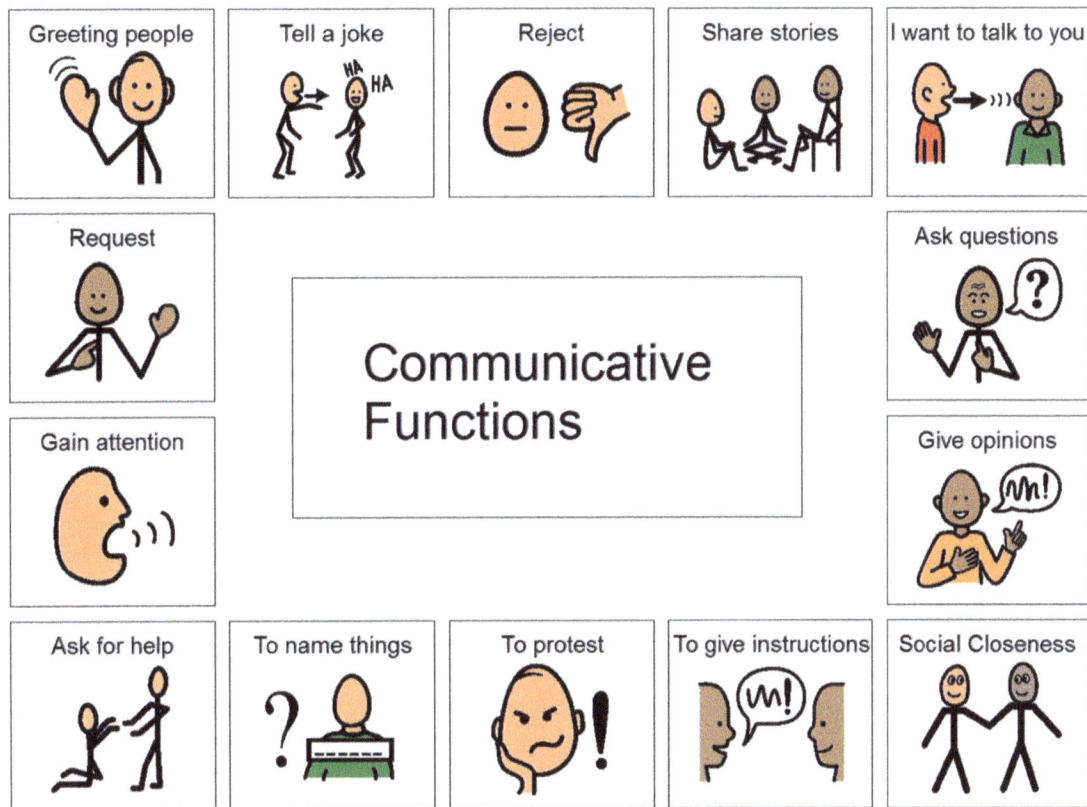

Figure 10.4 Communicative Functions poster.

Source: Created by the author using PCS symbols. PCS and Boardmaker are trademarks of Tobii Dynavox LLC. All rights reserved. Used with permission.

The Pragmatic Profile for AAC users

The Pragmatic Profile was adapted in 2017 by S. Martin, K. Small and R. Stevens, supported by the national charity, Ace Centre, which specialises in supporting AAC users. This adaptation became the Pragmatic Profile for AAC users and specifically focuses on referencing the use of AAC, unlike many of the other assessments available. This is an interview style tool where information is gathered by the interviewer from the team supporting the learner. There are a range of questions which link to different communicative functions and will help to profile the learner's language skills. Some examples of those interview questions are displayed here:

> 4.3
>
> Requesting cessation
>
> **If [name] wanted you to stop doing something or wanted to finish an activity, what would s/he do?**
>
> Answers could include. but are not limited to:
>
> *Cry*
> *Use a body movement or gesture [describe] vocalise*
> *Look at you with facial expression to say 'no' use AAC resource, e.g. to say 'stop' other? – please describe*
>
> 4.4
>
> Requesting assistance
>
> **If [name] needs help with something [e.g. to unfasten a lap belt, unwrap an item of food], what does s/he do?**

> Answers could include, but are not limited to:
> Cry
> Use a body movement or gesture [describe] vocalise
> Look at you with facial expression to say 'no' use AAC resource, e.g. to say 'stop' other? – please describe
>
> 4.5
> <u>Requesting an object</u>
> **If [name] wants an object [e.g., a favourite toy, blanket], what does s/he do?**
> Answers could include but are not limited to:
> Cry
> Use a body movement or gesture [describe] vocalise
> Look at you with facial expression to say 'no' use AAC resource, e.g. to say 'stop' other? – please describe
>
> 4.6
> <u>Response to direct request for action</u>
> **If you give [name] an instruction [e.g. 'move your arm [or other body part]', or' choose which book you want'], how does she respond?**
> Answers could include but are not limited to:
> Cry
> Use a body movement or gesture [describe] vocalise
> Look at you with facial expression to say 'no' use AAC resource, e.g. to say 'stop' other? – please describe

Each of these questions relate to different types of communicative functions. Once you have collated answers from the interview, answers next can be mapped onto the tables displayed. These highlight a clear profile of the learner's language skills in relation to the pragmatics of language and what tools they currently use to communicate.

Figure 10.5 is a sample of the summary sheet at the front of the document where the person who conducted the interview can check boxes which relate to the different communicative functions. Then, they identify through this document if that communicative function is utilised, may be utilised, is not utilised or is not applicable. It also has a box to check if it would be appropriate to set a target around developing skills in using this communicative function.

This chart (Figure 10.6) gives a clear overview of the different communication methods that a learner is currently using to convey those communicative functions, for example unaided by using eye pointing, body movement, vocalisation or verbal words and gestures, or by employing aided language using AAC. Another key part to the Overview of Communication Methods is that it also allows it to be documented whether the learner's communication of the different communicative functions can be understood for 'all' or familiar only 'FO'. This could also guide you on target setting, as a learner may be able to communicate a wide range of language functions, but if they are only understood by familiar communication partners this could prove to be limiting for them, as they will likely incur many communication breakdowns. This could have a negative effect on their mental health, especially if they have been used to everyone understanding them and then move settings and suddenly, they cannot communicate effectively with anyone.

The full Pragmatics Profile tool is freely downloadable from the charity Ace Centre at www.acecentre.org.uk/resources/pragmatics-profile-people-use-aac

The Affective Communication Assessment

The Affective Communication Assessment (ACA) is a tool to profile the different communication given by a learner who is still working at a pre-intentional language level. These learners are typically functioning at Piaget's Sensori Motor phase of cognitive development as detailed in Figure 10.7:

Contents Page / Summary Sheet

Part A: Establishing context & motivation

1

1.1	Likes
1.2	Dislikes
1.3	Key people
1.4	Key places

Part B: Reasons to communicate & reactions to communication

		Does this	May do this	Does not do this	Not applicable	Potential target
2	**Gaining attention for communication**					
2.1	Interest in interaction					
2.2	Gaining an individual's attention					
2.3	Understanding of gesture					
2.4	Gaining attention to prepare for an interaction					
3	**Attention directing**					
3.1	Drawing attention to self					
3.2	Drawing attention to an event or action					
3.3	Drawing attention to an object					
3.4	Drawing attention to other people					
4	**Requesting**					
4.1	Requesting a person					
4.2	Requesting recurrence					
4.3	Requesting cessation					
4.4	Requesting assistance					
4.5	Requesting an object					
4.6	Responding to a direct request for action					
4.7	Requesting an event or action					
4.8	Requesting information					
4.9	Responding to a request for information					
4.10	Requesting confirmation of information					
4.11	Understanding indirect requests					
5	**Rejecting**					
5.1	Rejecting a person					
5.2	Rejecting an object					
5.3	Rejecting an event or action or task					
5.4	Rejecting assistance					
5.5	Protesting					
5.6	Responding to 'no'					
5.7	Negotiating					
5.8	Responding to negotiation					

Figure 10.5 Contents Page/Summary Sheet.

Source: Created by the Ace Centre https://acecentre.org.uk/resources/pragmatics-profile-people-use-aac

The Affective Communication Assessment is a tool where observations can be recorded to look for consistent responses to stimuli, so communication partners can begin to map language onto those communicative behaviours (attributing meaning as discussed in the chapter on modelling). For example, a child consistently turning their head away when presented with a banana to communicate rejection of the banana. Making these observations can help educators and the wider team working with the learner to identify what behaviours are consistent, and what these behaviours may be communicating. The steps in this approach for establishing intentional communication, outlined by Coupe O'Kane and Goldbart (1998), are summarised below:

Methods of communication chart

*FO = Understood by familiar only
All = Understood by all

		Uses AAC resource: single words	Uses AAC resource: sentence or phrase	Eye pointing, eye contact		Body movement		Vocalisation, sound, word or word approximation		Sign		Gesture		Facial expression		Other
				FO*	ALL	FO	ALL	FO	ALL	FO	ALL	FO	ALL	FO	ALL	
1	**Context and motivation**															
1.1	Shows likes															
1.2	Shows dislikes															
2	**Gaining attention**															
2.1	Interest in interaction															
2.4	Gaining attention to prepare for an interaction															
3	**Drawing attention**															
3.1	... to self															
3.2	... to an event or action															
3.3	... to an object															
3.4	... to other people															
4	**Requesting**															
4.1	... a person															
4.2	... recurrence															
4.3	... cessation															
4.4	... assistance															
4.5	... an object															
4.6	Response to direct request for action															
4.7	... an event or action															
4.8	... information															
4.9	Responding to a request for information															
4.10	... confirmation of information															

Figure 10.6 Methods of communication chart.

Source: Created by the Ace Centre (https://acecentre.org.uk/resources/pragmatics-profile-people-use-aac).

Stage label	Approx. age (in months)	Cognitive, semantic and/or symbolic development
First habits	0-1	Infants engage mainly in reflex exercise, sucking, rooting and selective looking..
Primary circular reactions	1-4	When a baby does something with their body e.g. thumb-sucking, that they find pleasureable, they learn to repeat the action. Early undifferentiated schemes include looking, holding looking and mouthing.
Secondary circular reactions	4-8	When a baby does somethiung external to themselves that they find pleasureable, they learn to repeat the action. Fore example,
Coordination of secondary schemes	8-12	A baby's cognitive roles expand. Babies' use of familiar objects becomes more conventional. Goals identified before starting an activity (cognitive intentionality is fully established). Semantic roles to be conveyed.
Tertiary circular reactions	12-18	Babies demonstrate use of tools and new ways of achieving ends through experimentation. They show relational play before engaging in self-pretend play. Babies begin to use their first words, organised by semantic role.
Beginnings of thought	18-24	Toddlers predict cause and effect relationships. They show decentred pretend play, before sequenced pretend play. Complex gestures before two-word utterances, with increasing syntatic development,

Figure 10.7 Cognitive, semantic and symbolic development in Piaget's sensori-motor period.
Source: Created by the author.

First of all, a variety of stimuli are presented to the pupil and their observable responses to each are noted. These stimuli may be auditory, visual, tactile, gustatory or olfactory or a complex combination of these, such as human contact, specific sounds, tastes of specific foods, bright disco lights, and so on. The pupil must be given time to respond to each stimulus and a provisional interpretation of the meaning of the pupil's responses – vocalisations, facial expressions and/or body actions – has to be made in each case.

The next step involves representing those stimuli that evoked the pupil's strongest responses. Checks are made for the consistency of the pupil's responses and the behaviours that may be interpreted as 'like' or 'dislike' are identified.

The final step is to actually teach the pupil that behaving in certain ways will have an effect on the people who are doing these things to him or her. Situations are engineered which are known to evoke specific potentially communicative behaviour, i.e., the behaviour that can be said to communicate emotional reactions to the stimuli. When potentially communicative behaviour has been evoked, the teacher responds to the pupil's behaviour in a relevant and consistent way as though the pupil is intentionally communicating. If the pupil's behaviour indicates 'like', the interesting or pleasing item or activity is presented again. If the pupil's behaviour indicates 'dislike' the item or activity is stopped or withdrawn immediately. The assumption is that after sufficient experiences of this nature the pupil will come to realise that they can behave in ways that communicate desires or rejection of things or activities. In such interactions are sown the seeds of simple communication and choice making by many pupils.

Assessment takes the form of noting and recording responses to a range of planned experiences. For these individuals their responses and signs can be difficult to identify and interpret, particularly for adult who are less familiar. The outcome should be records of typical like and dislike behaviours in response to each type of experience.

http://complexneeds.org.uk/modules/Module-2.4-Assessment-monitoring-and-evaluation/All/m08p020b.html

---

The Affective Communication Assessment was developed as a way of recording observations of how pupils respond when given systematic presentations of a selection of stimuli, for example tastes, touches and smells. The supporting team can use this to record their findings and begin profiling the learners pre-intentional communication.

Once a student has been profiled, the information needs to be documented. There are numerous ways to do this, from communication passports to tick sheets and visual target displays. The

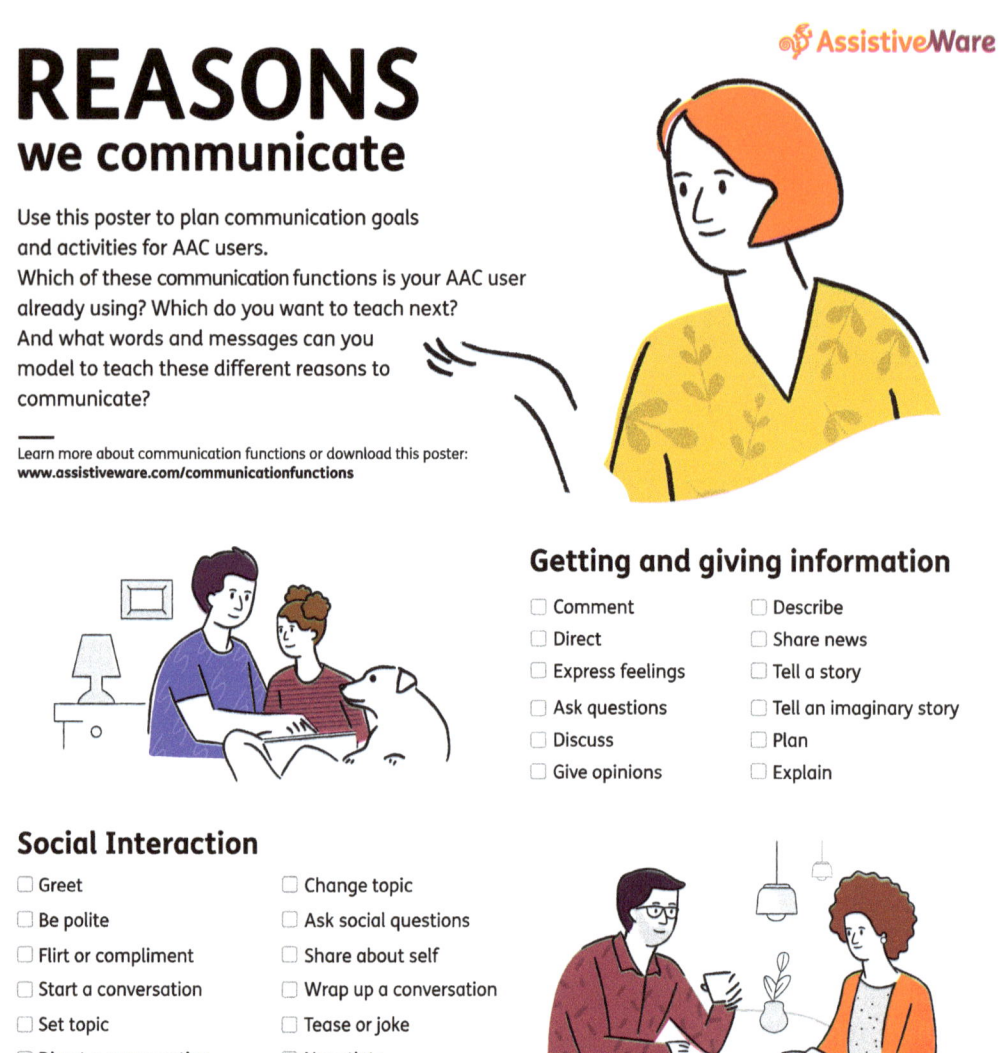

Figure 10.8 Reasons we communicate poster.

Source: www.assistiveware.com ©2019 AssistiveWare BV. All rights reserved. Symbols © 2019 SymbolStix, LLC.

most important thing is that everyone is consistent in understanding the learner's communication, and the team can identify what communicative functions the learner is currently expressing. Then the team can start to apply consistent language to those communicative functions, such as core words. Figure 10.8 is a useful checklist for mapping a learner in relation to communicative functions. It is downloadable from the AssistiveWare website.

Visual displays in the classroom profiling the communication that learners use, and their next steps will help the class team and other staff working with the learner to understand the learner's expressive language level. This will support staff in modelling aided language at an appropriate level.

By looking at typical language development we can now mirror this with the use of aided language. Language is learnt through natural interaction, not staged interventions. Those interactions are meaningful and in true contexts. There is no testing or expectations on the learner to communicate a specific answer – after all, communication needs to be autonomous.

Some children will, however, need more direct instruction. Not in the form of a once-a-week communication lesson. Rather, communication partners being explicit about why they are communicating with the learner. An example of an AAC tool that does this is PODD – Pragmatic Organised Dynamic Display (Figure 10.9).

The Pragmatic Organisation of language in a dynamic display means that the reason why we are communicating is always the starting point for the interaction. Below are a list of pragmatic starters displayed in the PODD communication system.

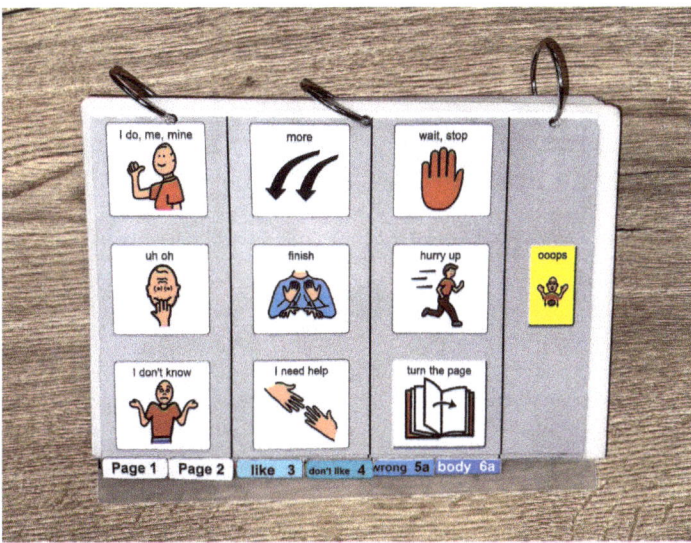

Figure 10.9 Spiral bound book with 15 symbols displayed.

Source: Photographed by the author.

- I'm asking a question
- I'm telling you something
- I'm telling a story
- I have an idea
- Let's pretend
- I want to show you something
- I want
- Let's go
- Do something
- I like this
- I don't like this
- Something's wrong

When thinking about reasons why we communicate with others, we can see that this system covers a wide range of those communicative functions. The PODD system in paper-based format often relies on the communication partner to turn to the page number selected on the initial page and navigate through the book as instructed by the learner.

Pragmatic Organised Dynamic Display system, PODD, is explicit about teaching those communicative functions to learners who need support with language development. A speech and language therapist assessment would ascertain if an AAC system that is pragmatically organised, would be suitable for your learner. In the absence of having access to specific AAC, such as PODD, or the absence of having a speech and language therapy assessment, communication partners can adapt their communication partner skills and be explicit with the learner about the communicative functions they are using in the interaction. For example, 'Mike, I'm asking you a question: What is your dog called?' Or 'Mike, I'm telling you something: My dog is called Archie.' The more we teach these communicative functions, be that through attributing meaning to core words or using pragmatically organised AAC, the more communicative functions a learner will be able to use and, consequently, the more their language skills will develop. This will in turn help them to achieve the desired goal of autonomous communication, which we know will allow them to take their place in society and help them to express their true self, which can only promote positive mental health and happiness.

Conclusion

Communication is so much more than requesting and answering closed questions. From delving into this chapter, we can see that those communicative functions are so important. They are the reasons why we communicate and our motivation for the interaction in the first place. By looking at how children's language has developed in a natural context it is clear that the pragmatics of language, the purpose for the interaction is fundamental.

There are lots of low-cost resources available to support the development of a learner's-use of aided language for language development. The next chapter will signpost to some of these, offering printable resources for your classroom.

Bibliography

Autism CRC. (2020). *Interventions for children on the autism spectrum*. [online] Available at: www.autismcrc.com.au/interventions-evidence

Bondy, A. and Frost, L. (2001). The Picture Exchange Communication System. *Behavior Modification*, 25(5), p. 728.

Dewart, H. and Summers, S. (1995). *The pragmatics profile of everyday communication skills in children*. Windsor: Nfer-Nelson.

Martin, S., Small, K. and Stevens, R. (2017). The Pragmatics Profile for People who use AAC (First Published 26 Sep 2017). Available at: https://acecentre.org.uk/resources/pragmatics-profile-people-use-aac/

Piaget, J. (1936). *Origins of intelligence in the child*. London: Routledge & Kegan Paul.

Porter, G. (2018). *Pragmatic organisation dynamic display communication books: Introductory workshop*. Melb: Cerebral Palsy Education Centre.

Shkedy, G., Shkedy, D. and Sandoval-Norton, A.H. (2021). Long-term ABA Therapy Is Abusive: A Response to Gorycki, Ruppel, and Zane. *Advances in Neurodevelopmental Disorders*, 5, pp.126–134.

11 Low Cost, Effective Resources

Attributes of Paper-based Resources

Paper-based resources may have different attributes that are worth considering when choosing what's relevant for your learner. These include:

- How words and concepts are represented, for example, using graphic symbols or text.
- How the resource is created, for example using resources such as paper, cardboard, ring folders, laminated pages, or rip proof paper, which are all available within a school setting.
- Whether the resource requires the use of symbol-generating software to create the resource, for example Boardmaker and Communicate in Print.
- How easy the resource is to customise and consider how much vocabulary to use, which will impact on the weight of the resources, so you can make resources lighter as necessary.
- How easy it is to attach pages together, for example through use of spiral binding.
- How the communication partner will facilitate the communication, for example navigating through pages or acting as the voice output.

Positives of Paper-based Resources

Paper-based resources have many positives, which make them suitable for learners and meet their communication needs without the need for electronic communication aids. These include:

- Paper-based resources are robust, reliable low cost and quick to create.
- Paper-based resources can be used to support the learner in using a range of communicative functions, for example, requesting, commenting, expressing opinions, and rejecting.
- Paper-based resources lay a good foundation and introduction to aided language/AAC, allowing the learner to develop communicative competence before considering electronic communication aids, for example operational, linguistic, social, and strategic competence (Light, 1989).
- Paper-based resources can be easy for communication partners to pick up and use with the learner and can be used across environments; for example, laminated resources could be used in the swimming pool, bath, transport, and during personal care, where the use of an electronic communication aid would not be accessible (water and technology does not mix!).
- Paper-based resources also do not run out of battery or charge, unlike electronic communication aids. Paper-based resources, even when a learner has an electronic communication aid, are necessary due to the risk of the electronic communication aid failing and leaving the learner without a voice.
- Paper-based resources can be duplicated to ensure they are readily available in all settings. For example, having a copy of the learner's communication book both at home and school. However, it is important to consider consistency. The two copies must match each other, with the same symbols laid out in the same manner.
- Paper-based resources can be easy to navigate. Due to the navigation required to locate vocabulary, electronic communication aids can be overwhelming, particularly at first for the learner and communication partner. Technology can sometimes cause a barrier for those learners and communication partners who are not used to using technology in their daily life.
- Paper-based resources can be quicker and more efficient as the communication partner is able to pick up on the learner's non-verbal cues, for example gesture, body language, and vocalisations. If a learner points to a specific toy and is exhibiting positive body language

and vocalisations, this can be interpreted as the learner liking the object. The communication partner can also verify with the learner as to whether what they are interpreting and communicating is correct, and whether they have meant to choose a given symbol, or whether this is a miss-hit. This alleviates any misunderstandings.
- Paper-based resources can evolve organically, with extra vocabulary being easy to add – for example you can just print out the new page for a communication book and off you go!

Barriers to Implementing Paper-based Resources

Despite the positive impact of paper-based resources, you may still face colleagues or parents who feel there are barriers to using these. It would be worthwhile to have conversations around the implementation of paper-based resources prior to introducing these to the learner, ensuring they have a positive impact.

These barriers may include individuals feeling that:

- Electronic is better than paper-based.
- Resources do not meet the learner's communication needs.
- Voice output is the desired goal, and the learner is unable to communicate without this being facilitated by an adult.

Due to these barriers, resources can be modelled less, and staff may not support their implementation. This leads to the learner being less motivated to use the resource, which in turn leads to the learner not having consistent access to the resource throughout and across settings.

Due to these challenges, it can often be helpful to include with the resource brief written instructions on how to use it to build colleague's confidence and understanding of the importance of the resource. It is also important to identify a key person, or people to be responsible for keeping the resource up to date and adding any new vocabulary.

Skills Developed by using Paper-based Resources

Learners acquire a wealth of skills when using paper-based resources. Some of these are listed below:

- Understanding the purpose of communication aid is to share thoughts with others.
- Developing an understanding of what the symbols represent.
- Developing of skills to access AAC, for example learning to isolate a finger to point to relevant symbols.
- Understanding how to use different word types to communicate a range of language functions, aside from requesting nouns, for example using verbs and adjectives.
- Understanding how to categorise words into categories for example places, food and drink, and people to easily access relevant vocabulary without having to trawl through pages.
- Developing the skills to repair communication when the communication partner has not understood their message, for example using AAC to augment speech when speech is not intelligible. Strategies can include: *'it begins with ...'*, *'it is like ...'*, *'it is a place'*.
- Supporting language development, for example creating sentence strings by combining symbols together and supporting sentence construction, for example creating more complex sentences than the learner is able to communicate verbally.

Considerations for Creating Paper-based Resources

When creating paper-based resources there are some points to consider. These include:

- How the learner accesses the resource?
- Making sure the resource is organised appropriately.
- Supporting the development of language skills through the layout of the resource.
- Whether text, symbols or both will be used within the resource to represent vocabulary?

Personalisation

For the resource to be used successfully, it is important to consider personalising the resource to make it meaningful and motivating for the learner. The language available has to represent what the learner wishes to talk about, for example a learner may have a keen interest in *Thomas the Tank Engine*.

Consider:

- What environments is the learner communicating in?
- When is the learner communicating?
- Who is the learner communicating with?
- Which people are important to them?
- What is the purpose of the learner's interaction?
- What is the learner doing?
- What activities does the learner enjoy?

Discussion Point!

- Consider a learner in your classroom who uses aided language/AAC.
- Looking at the questions above, what core and fringe vocabulary would this learner need?
- Do you have enough vocabulary available to enable the learner to use a range of language functions? For example, commenting, asking questions, negating.

Symbol Sets

The different symbol sets have been discussed earlier in this book, so it is worth referring back to it for a deeper dive into the different options. When considering the symbol set to use on a paper-based resource, weigh up which symbol set would be most appropriate for the learner. Some schools use the same symbol set as a whole school for all resources. The main symbol sets are:

- Widgit symbols
- PCS symbols
- Symbol Stix symbols

Although some of the paper-based resources do not require access to symbol generating software, in order to make personalisations many schools use software such as Boardmaker and Communicate in Print to use either PCS or Widgit symbols. Sadly, these are paid-for software, so not all schools have it. If this is the case within your school, reach out to other local schools in the area, for example specialist schools who may be able to support you in creating resources.

Organisation of Resources

It is important when considering making your own resources that you think about how you are going to organise vocabulary to make it most easily accessible for the learner. Things to consider include:

Are you going to organise the vocabulary pragmatically, taxonomically, or schematically?
- Pragmatically organised – based on communicating the function or reason why the learner is communicating first; for example: 'Something's wrong', 'I have a question', 'I want something'.
- Taxonomically organised – based on categories, for example food and drink.
- Schematically organised – based on context of location, where symbols represent the scene or context, for example, the kitchen.

Are you going to consider colour-coding the resource?
Many aided language resources follow the Fitzgerald key (1929). The colour coding for this is seen below:
- Blue – Adjectives
- Green – Verbs
- Yellow – Pronouns
- Orange – Nouns
- White – Conjunctions
- Pink – Prepositions, social words
- Purple – Questions
- Brown – Adverbs
- Red – Important function words negation, emergency words
- Grey – Determiners

Amount of vocabulary per page? Number of pages in the resource? How is the vocabulary going to be laid out?

Access

How is the learner going to access the resource?

- Does the learner experience any visual difficulties which will affect their ability to visually access the resource? Does this have an impact on the number of symbols used, their sizing and how they are spaced on the page?
- Does the learner have difficulties which will make it challenging to point?
- Is the learner able to directly access the resource?
- Does the learner need assistance accessing the resource, for example through partner-assisted scanning?

There are a range of different paper-based resources to download and use with your learners.

Type of resource	Name of resource	Who is the resource created by	Format of resource	Description of resource	Cost of the resource	Useful links to the resource
Communication book Three communication boards with various icons on a wooden floor.	PODD (Pragmatically Organised Dynamic Display)	Gayle Porter	A range of layouts available to cater for different access methods and level of language development	Arranged pragmatically, based on the function or reason of communication	£199 for the software containing the templates, however you will need Boardmaker or Mind Express symbol generating software to download and use the templates. Alternative access templates are an additional £199	To purchase: www.inclusive.co.uk/podd-p6023 www.inclusive.com/uk/podd-alternative-access-a4-version.html
Communication book An open communication book in a binder. The left page has icons for phrases like I, me, mine, more, again, look, see. The right page depicts actions like playing computer games and singing.	Developing and Using a Communication Book	Ace Centre	Category based, with consistent core on each page alongside specific fringe vocabulary. Guide contains 5 stages to support language development.	A guidebook in how to create core and fringe based communication books	£50 for the guidebook. The templates can be downloaded for free. You will need the symbol generating software Boardmaker or Communicate in Print to download and use the templates.	To purchase: https://acecentre.org.uk/resources/developing-using-communication-book

108 *Low Cost, Effective Resources*

Type of resource	Name of resource	Who is the resource created by	Format of resource	Description of resource	Cost of the resource	Useful links to the resource
Communication book A spiral book on a stand, divided into sections with different colored backgrounds. It contains various icons representing everyday activities, emotions, and objects for non-verbal communication. Created by Ace Centre www.acecentre.org.uk	Look 2 Talk	Ace Centre	Category based with consistent core vocabulary alongside fringe vocabulary. Guide contains 5 stages to support language development. Uses eye pointing to access the communication book.	A guidebook in how to create a core and fringe vocabulary book which can be access through eye pointing	Free to view guidance online and download templates to be used in symbol generating software Boardmaker	Download from: https://acecentre.org.uk/resources/look2talk/ Easel can be purchased separately from: www.ability-world.com/a4-communication-easel-5395-p.asp
Communication book A colorful grid communication aid with words and symbols for pronouns, verbs, adjectives, prepositions, and common phrases like what, where, who, and so on. Image courtesy of Liberator Ltd. All rights reserved. Widgit Symbols © Widgit Software Ltd 2002–2023 www.widgit.com	Liberator Paper-Based Support Books	Liberator	Paper copies of Liberator vocabularies to make into a flipbook with a core page and tabbed fringe pages	Ready-made paper-based communication books to use based on Liberator's vocabularies on electronic communication aids, including easyChat Core (with Widgit, PCS and SymbolStix) with 45, 60 and 84 locations, LAMP Words for Life, easyChat Phrases (PCS), WordPower (with PCS and SymbolStix) 42, 60 and 108 locations	Free – PDF documents	Download from: www.liberator.co.uk/resources/low-tech-support-books

Communication book	TD Snap Core First Communication books	Tobii Dynavox	Communication book templates available in two sizes – 6x6 and 7x9. Includes core words, Quickfires and popular topics.	Ready-made paper-based communication books based on TD Snap Core First vocabulary on an electronic communication aid. Available in different languages.	Free – PDF documents	Download from: https://uk.tobiidynavox.com/products/core-first-communication-boards
A core first communication book with core words each paired with a symbol. Words include what, who, where, and actions like want, can, go. *PCS and Boardmaker are trademarks of Tobii Dynavox LLC. All rights reserved. Used with permission*						
Communication book	Super Core communication book	Smartbox	Communication book arranged with tabs and consistent access to core vocabulary. Provided on rip-proof paper, in a folder and carry strap.	Paper-based communication book based on Super Core50 vocabulary available on electronic communication aids	£295. Template pages can be downloaded from the Smartbox website	To purchase: https://thinksmartbox.com/product/super-core-communication-book/
A colorful communication board divided into core, activities, and topics. Some of the icons with words read, who, what, why, again, finish, and more. Smartbox, creators of Grid AAC software						

Type of resource	Name of resource	Who is the resource created by	Format of resource	Description of resource	Cost of the resource	Useful links to the resource
Communication boards. A tabular diagram with 30 labeled grids with their associated symbols is as follows. Like, won't, get, make, more, not go, look, turn, help, he, open, do, put, same, you, she, that, up, some, it, here, in, on, can, where, who, when, and stop. University of North Carolina at Chapel Hill, The Center for Literacy and Disability Studies, www.project-core.com.	Project Core	Center for Literacy and Disability Studies.	Core word boards. Different layouts to support a range of access methods, levels of vision, cognitive abilities, etc. Each resource is available in PCS, Widgit and Symbolstix. Additional lessons are available to support learning regarding core word implementation.	Communication boards based on 36 universal core words. Different layouts and access methods available e.g. 4, 6, 9 and 36 symbols per page, high contrast symbols and eye gaze access. CAD files to can be downloaded to create 3D symbols.	Free	Download from: www.project-core.com/communication-systems/
Communication boards. A tabular diagram with 30 labeled grids titled core words with their associated symbols is as follows. I, me, my, mine, More, look, question, you and yours, want, make, play, she and hers, different, big, it, go, have and has, bad, like, and not. Created by Ace Centre www.acecentre.org.uk	Ace Centre Communication Boards	Ace Centre	Individual symbol charts for different contexts e.g. core commenting charts, bubbles and art and crafts. Available in Widgit, PCS and SymbolStix. Available in different layouts for different access methods, including direct access, colour encoded eye pointing, and high contrast. These can be customised through the Ace Centre website.	Symbols Core word charts to be used in a range of activities.	Free	Download from: https://acecentre.org.uk/product-category/symbol-charts/

Low Cost, Effective Resources

Communication boards A tabular diagram with 28 labeled grids with their associated symbols is as follows. I want, names, chat, help, scroll, I need, drinks, food, feelings, places, about me, animals, body, toys, read, school, clear all, time, social, and more. Image courtesy of Liberator Ltd. All rights reserved. Symbols included are SymbolStix ® Copyright © 2023 SymbolStix, LLC. All rights reserved. Used with Permission	Liberator manual boards	Liberator	Individual pages for given vocabulary's top core page. Available in corresponding symbols sets, including Widgit, Boardmaker, and SymbolStix	Manual boards of the front page of Liberator vocabularies including: UNITY and LAMP words for life easyChat Core easyChat Phrases easyChat Spell easyChat Words WordPower for Accent Word Scanner WordPower for Chat devices MultiChat15 Communication Journey Aphasia My Core My quick chat	Free	Download from: www.liberator.co.uk/resources/manual_boards
Communication boards A tabular diagram with 35 labeled grids with their associated symbols is as follows. Who, what, why, again, finish, want, see, now, that, open, it, go, stop, in, on, put, you or your, help, like, not, here, choose, hurt, different, play, and turn. Smartbox, creators of Grid AAC software	Super Core Pages	Smartbox	Single and double-sided communication boards suitable for direct access. These mirror Super Core 30 or 50, available in Widgit, PCS and SymbolStix	Core word manual boards to match the top page of Super Core 30 and 50.	Free	Download from: https://thinksmartbox.com/news/resources/get-started-with-super-core/

112 Low Cost, Effective Resources

Type of resource	Name of resource	Who is the resource created by	Format of resource	Description of resource	Cost of the resource	Useful links to the resource
Communication boards	Super Core Learning Grids	Smartbox	Communication boards based on Super Core Learning Grids, available on 12 and 20 locations, available in Widgit, PCS and SymbolStix	Individual context specific communication boards linked to Super Core Learning Grids, e.g. eating and drinking, playing ball, crafts	Free	Download from: https://thinksmartbox.com/news/resources/get-started-with-super-core/
Communication boards	ProloQuo and ProloQuo2Go manual boards	Assistive Ware	Communication boards to mimic the top pages of ProloQuo and ProloQuo2Go with an alphabet chart on the back	Manual communication boards for the core page of ProloQuo and ProloQuo2Go	Free	www.assistiveware.com/learn-aac/quick-communication-boards

A tabular diagram with 12 labeled grids titled ball with their associated symbols is as follows. Want, again, go, big, stop, throw, ball, little, more, bounce, roll, and up.

Smartbox, creators of Grid AAC software

A tabular diagram with 77 labeled grids with their associated symbols is as follows. I, can, will, who, not, need, to, all done, she, go, take, for, it, there, bad, think, off, some, eat, feelings, time, or, people, actions, and little words.

www.AssistiveWare.com ©2019
AssistiveWare BV. All rights reserved.
Symbols © 2019 SymbolStix, LLC

Points to Consider if Pointing is Difficult

Eye Pointing

Paper-based eye-pointing resources can be more successful than electronic communication aids accessed via eye gaze due to difficulties regarding the different cameras being able to pick up and read a learner's eyes, particularly when they have eye conditions such as nystagmus, or have a lot of involuntary movements. The eye gaze cameras do not always read a learner's eyes well when the learner wears glasses, and cameras are sensitive to light, with many not being able to be used in bright sunlight.

Alternatively, paper-based eye pointing resources are facilitated by a communication partner, who is able to verbally clarify whether they have read the learner's eyes correctly, which electronic communication aids are unable to do.

The use of an E-Tran frame is one example of a resource which can be used by learners who use eye pointing.

The E-Tran frame is positioned between the learner and communication partner. The learner can create messages by eye-pointing at relevant symbols or letters in given locations on the chart. E-Tran frames can often include colour encoding systems. For example, Figure 11.1 is an image for simple colour coding using a resource created by Ace Centre. If the learner wishes to say 'stop' they would first eye point to the group in the top left and then to the blue spot.

Johnathan Bryan (Figure 11.2), who set up the charity Teach Us Too and advocates all learners should be given the opportunity to read and write, uses an E-Tran frame to communicate. He has previously trialled electronic communication aids, but these did not pick up his eyes, whereas a communication partner was able to do so. Using the E-Tran frame he is a confident and efficient communicator, having written a book using this access method.

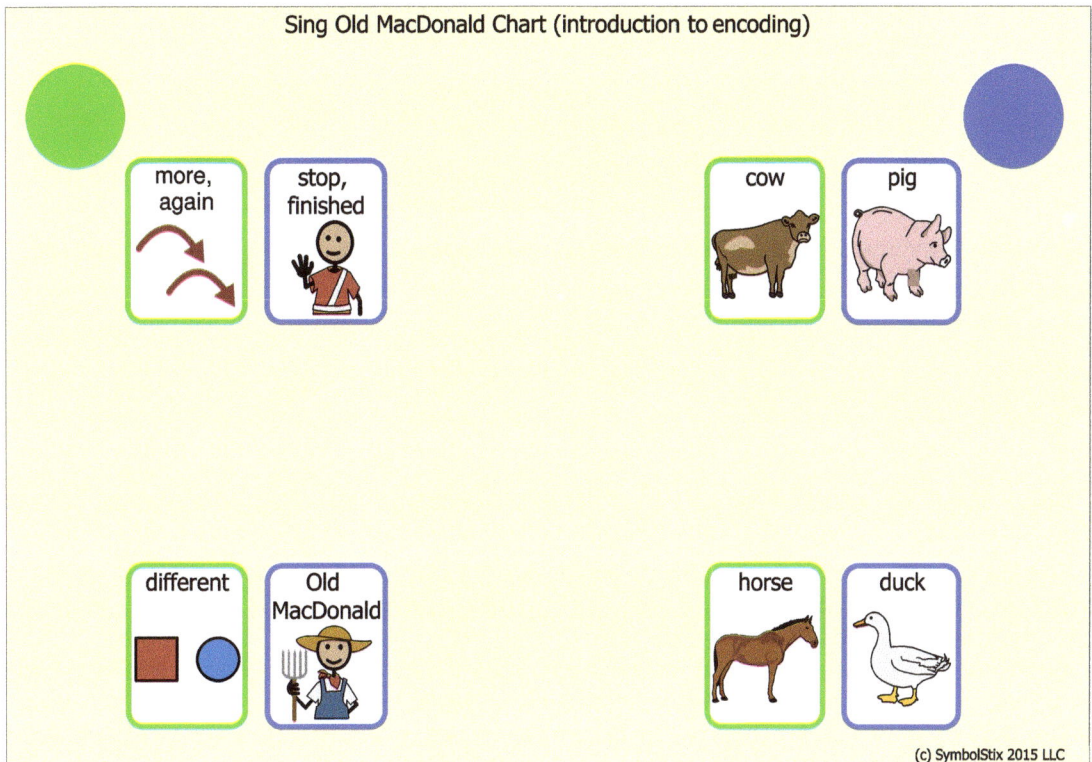

Figure 11.1 This image shows green and blue in each corner and words relating to farm animals.
Source: Created by Ace Centre www.acecentre.com

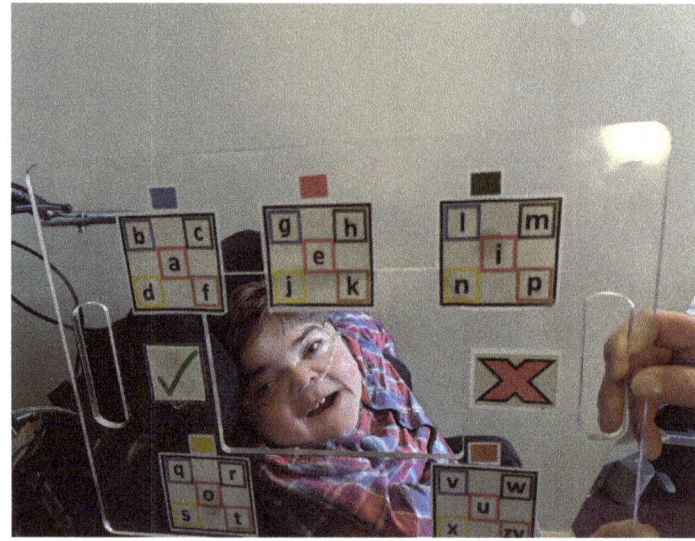

Figure 11.2 This image shows a young man using an eye pointing chart. Image from 'Teach Us Too'.
Source: Photograph provided by Chantal Bryan.

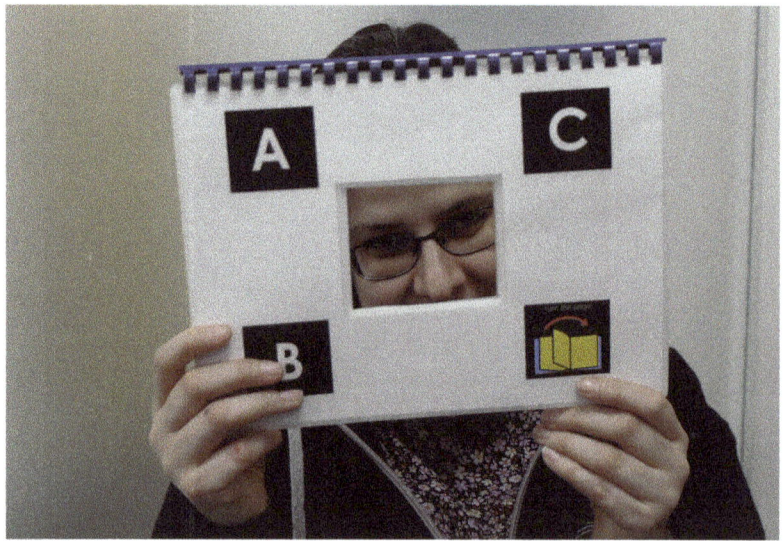

Figure 11.3 This image shows a woman holding a piece of paper with the letters a hole to look through.
Source: Photograph taken by the author.

Resources to Download:

Project Core have several examples on their website of four corner eye gaze universal core communication books with different symbols sets. Accessed here: www.project-core.com/4-corners/

The Centre of Literacy and Disability Studies have a range of 'alternative pencils', some of which are accessible via eye gaze (Figure 11.3). These can be accessed here: www.med.unc.edu/healthsciences/clds/alternative-pencils/

Ace Centre have also produced the resource *Look 2 Talk* which is a communication book accessed via eye pointing, with different stages to support language development and acquisition of eye pointing skills. This can be downloaded here: https://acecentre.org.uk/resources/look2talk A example demo page is shown here Figure 11.4.

To produce pages to use this resource, symbol generation software, for example Boardmaker and Communicate in Print is required, however Ace Centre also have resources which are downloadable to use without the need for symbol generating software. One example can be seen here (Figure 11.5): https://acecentre.org.uk/resources/listen-to-music-eye-pointing.

Low Cost, Effective Resources 115

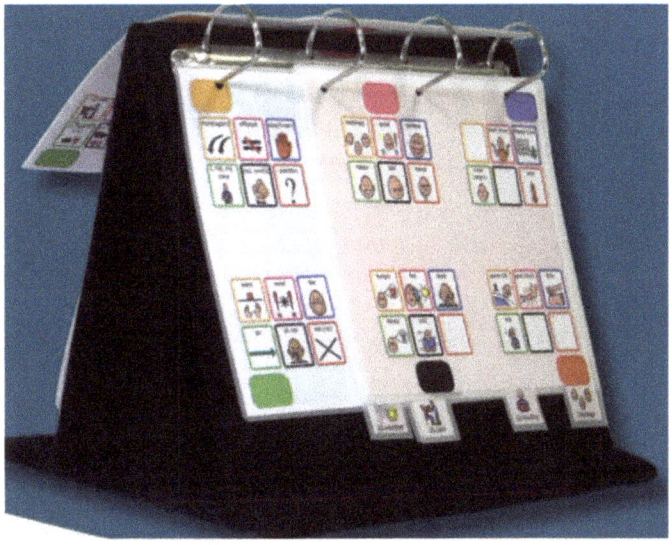

Figure 11.4 This image shows a Folder back, upright ring binder.

Source: Created by Ace Centre www.acecentre.com

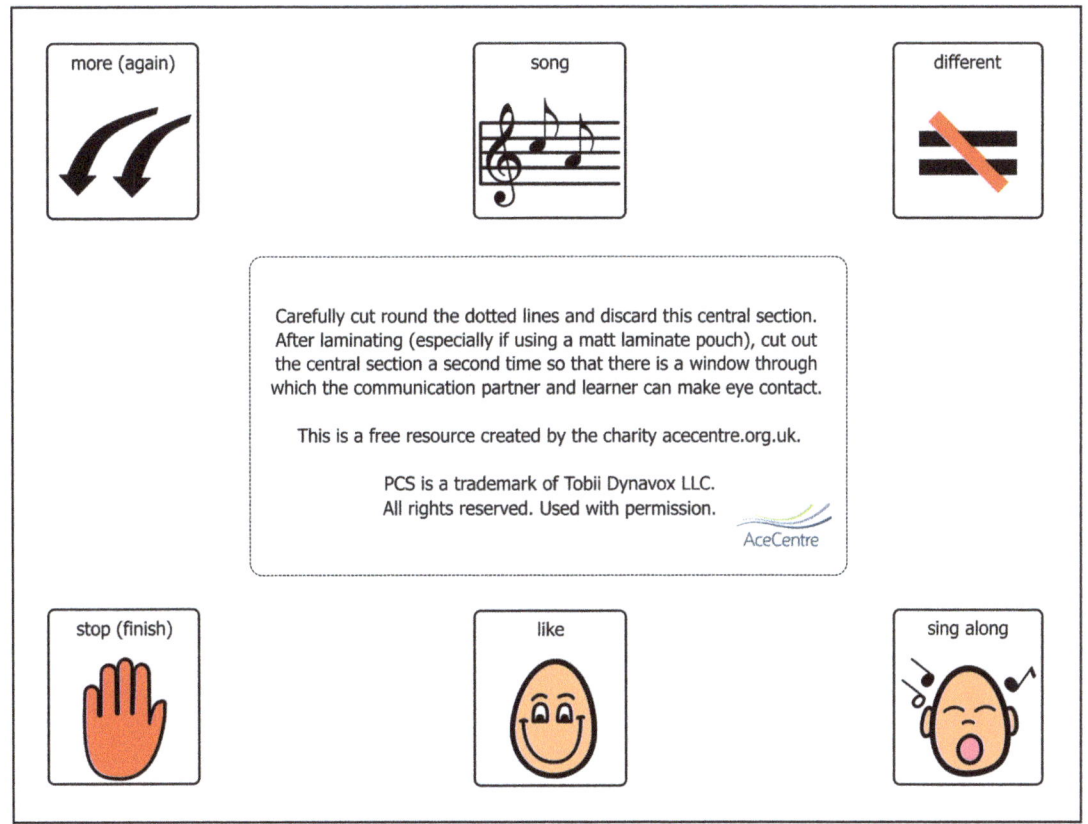

Figure 11.5 This image shows a chart with 6 symbols relating to singing.

Source: Created by Ace Centre www.acecentre.com

Patrick Joyce, in partnership with Ace Centre also created a *Speakbook*, which includes a series of paper-based E-Tran frames bound in a book.

An eye-link is another example of a paper-based resource which can be accessed through eye pointing (Figure 11.6). This is a transparent frame, which usually has letters displayed, which the communication partner holds between themselves and the learner. The learner will gaze to one letter/symbol at a time in order to construct a message or spell out a word. Barnsley hospital have an example of one available here with letters: www.barnsleyhospital.nhs.uk/assistive-technology/resource/eyelink-communication-boards/

The eye link can be used to develop eye pointing skills and making choices.

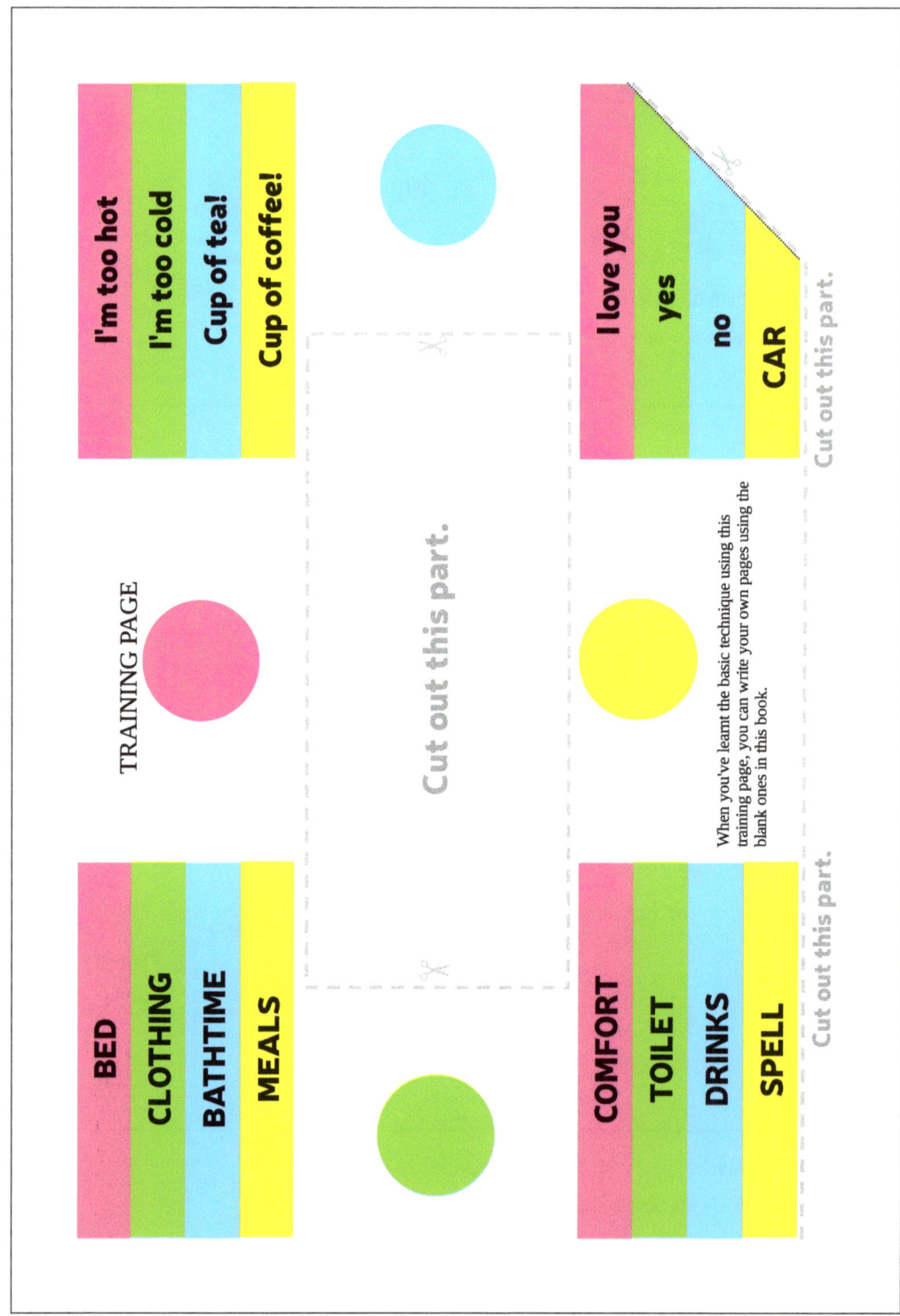

Figure 11.6 This image shows an image of a columns and dots which are pink, blue, green and yellow.

Source: Created by Ace Centre www.acecentre.com

Access to the Alphabet

For learners who are developing their literacy skills, consider whether alphabet, or spelling charts would be more appropriate for them than symbol charts. All learners should be given the opportunity to learn to read and write as 'no student is too anything to be able to read and write' (Yodder, 2000). A good place to start is to ensure all learners have access to the alphabet within their AAC system whether or not they are literate.

Spelling Charts

Spelling charts can be suitable for individuals who are literate or are developing literacy. They can be designed to accommodate an individual's access needs, including vision and hand function. They can be used with direct access, with partner-assisted scanning or with eye-pointing. They usually include all the letters of the alphabet, as well as some phrases in some instances. The layout of spelling charts can vary, however points to consider when choosing which symbol chart to use include:

- What access method is the learner going to use?
- What layout of the alphabet are they most familiar with?

Different layouts of spelling charts include:

- QWERTY layout is the most commonly used format, for example seen on keyboards.
- ABC layout is ordered according to the alphabet. This is often used for direct access, as well as partner-assisted scanning.
- AEIOU layout is used often when using partner-assisted scanning. Partner-assisted scanning will be covered in the supporting alternative access chapter later in this book.
- FREQUENCY layout is arranged so that the most frequently used letters are placed nearest the beginning and the least frequent letters are further away so will take longer to scan. This increases efficiency when using the spelling chart through scanning.
- FITALY layout is created for those learners who have reduced movement. This layout has the most common letters closer together so that the movement required to use the chart is reduced.

A range of different layouts are available on the Ace Centre website, which can be easily customised (Figure 11.7). You can access these here: https://acecentre.org.uk/resources/qwerty-2 Consider what size may be most appropriate for the learner, alongside making

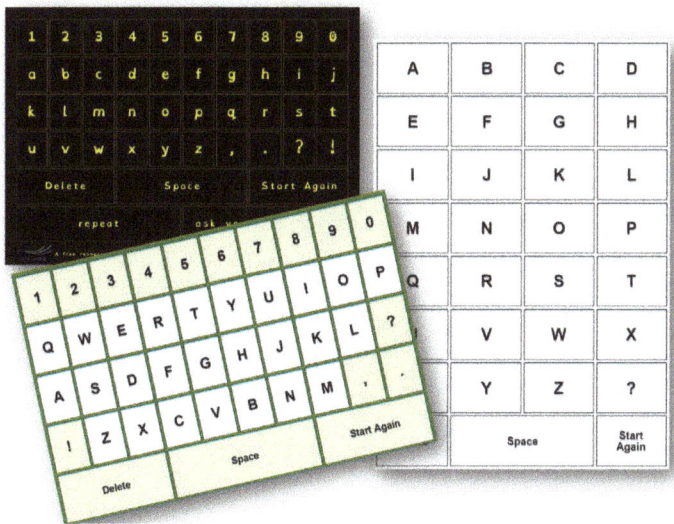

Figure 11.7 This image shows 3 different pages with the alphabet.

Source: Created by Ace Centre www.acecentre.com

changes to the resource yourself, for example changing the colour combination so it is more visually accessible.

When using spelling charts it is helpful to have a pen and paper handy to write down what the learner is saying, as it can be challenging to remember all the letters chosen to create a word.

Conclusion

This chapter shared a range of low-cost effective paper-based resources to support your learners who use aided language/AAC. These can be implemented with learners to support their language development and give them access to aided language. Due to financial constraints in schools, these are examples of how to implement aided language within the classroom without breaking the bank! Remember, a robust paper-based system can go everywhere with a learner and doesn't run out of charge. Due to this, it is advised to have a paper-based system alongside an electronic AAC device is your learner is using one.

The success of these resources is dependent on good communication partner skills by all those communicating with the learner. It is important that the learner has access to their AAC system and this is modelled to them to support them in getting their message across and continued language development.

Bibliography

Department for Education and Department of Health (2019). *Realising the potential of technology in education: A strategy for education providers and the technology industry*. Available at: https://assets.publishing.service.gov.uk/media/5ca360bee5274a77d479facc/DfE-Education_Technology_Strategy.pdf (Accessed: 14 January 2024)

Fitzgerald, E. (1929). *Straight language for the deaf: A system of instruction for deaf children.* Michigan: Edwards Brothers Inc.

Light, J. (1989). Toward a Definition of Communicative Competence for Individuals Using Augmentative and Alternative Communication Systems. *Augmentative and Alternative Communication*, 5(2), pp.137–144.

Yodder, D. (2000). *DJI-AbleNet literacy lecture*. ISAAC.

12 Communication Partner Skills

Who is Classed as a Communication Partner?

A communication partner is classed as anyone who interacts with the learner, from family and close friends to people in the community, for example, at the shop or café. Blackstone's circle of communication partners (1999) (Figure 12.1) identifies who are the most common to the least common communication partners for a learner. Within the different circles the communication partners will have varying understanding of the learners needs, thus interacting in a variety of ways. Close communication partners such as family will be able to pick up on the learner's body language and have a deeper understanding of how the learner communicates, whereas unfamiliar communication partners may not be able to tune into the learner's speech or pick up on their body language. Individuals may move between circles during a learner's lifetime, for example paid workers, or carers, may become life-long communication partners over time as they become more familiar with the learner and spend an increasing amount of time with them. The strategies used by the communication partners within each circle to support aided language will vary immensely due to the skill set of the communication partner and their understanding of aided language and how to support this effectively. It is essential that those communication partners who interact with the learner on a regular basis have the confidence, skills, knowledge and understanding to effectively support the learner.

What Will Communication Partners in Each Circle Benefit from?

- Lifelong communication partners:
  a. Learning a new way of communicating with the learner, learning, and teaching communication strategies they have not seen previously and have not implemented.
  b. Supporting the learner to identify why they may want to use aided language/AAC.
  c. Videoing other communication partners using AAC.

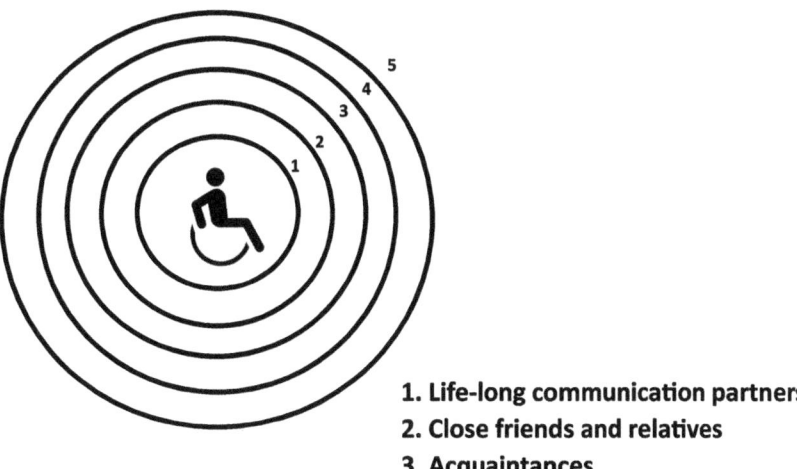

1. Life-long communication partners
2. Close friends and relatives
3. Acquaintances
4. Paid workers
5. Unfamiliar communication partners

Figure 12.1 Image of person in a wheelchair surrounded by five circles.

Source: Adapted from Blackstone's circle of communication partners (1999).

- d. Modelling from other communication partners using AAC, for example, other parents.
- e. Ongoing support regarding implementation of AAC.
- f. Ensuring the AAC system has adequate vocabulary, which has been personalised for the learner.
- g. Ensuring positive interactions with the learner.
- Close friends, relatives and acquaintances
    - a. Learning basic strategies to use to support interactions with the learner.
    - b. Providing written information regarding how to implement the learner's AAC system.
    - c. Modelling and guidance as to practice which will enable a change in behaviours for the learner.
- Paid workers
    - a. Providing models of the learner using their AAC system with experienced communication partners.
    - b. Experiencing interacting with the learner using their AAC system.
    - c. Training in how to use the learner AAC system, for example how their system is organised.
    - d. Providing a copy of the learner's AAC system (if possible) to enable the communication partner to practise using the learner's AAC system when they are not present to become more familiar.
    - e. Support from a communication partner who has more experience using the learner's AAC system to enable the communication partner to become more confident when interacting with the learner.
- Paid workers as a facilitator
    - a. Experience communication partner facilitating the interaction, assisting the communication partner and learner.
    - b. Having less of an active role during interactions with the learner.
    - c. Structuring the environment in order to support communication, for example considering appropriate strategies to use with the learner.
    - d. Enabling diverse and meaningful opportunities for communication between the communication partner and learner.
    - e. Prompting the learning only when necessary.
    - f. Modelling relevant communication strategies.
    - g. Verbally describing what they are doing.
    - h. Supporting the learner to problem solve and communicate their desired message.
    - i. Providing verbal hints and observations, supporting the learner to recognise patterns of their AAC system.
    - j. Making suggestions regarding what the learner could communicate in a given situation.
    - k. Providing a 'safety net' so that interactions are successful, preventing and solving any communication breakdowns which arise.
- Unfamiliar partners
    - a. Becoming communication partners incidentally.
    - b. Rarely automatically interacting with the learner.
    - c. Helping the learner to provide an explanation regarding their AAC system (if possible, or this can be facilitated by a familiar communication partner).
    - d. Familiar communication partners providing information for unfamiliar partners regarding what they should/shouldn't communicate with the learner.

Communication partners who are new to using aided language and AAC can often become overwhelmed. More experienced communication partners, as identified in Blackstone's circle of communication partners (1999), can offer advice and guidance to support the learner's communication. Binger C. and Kent-Walsh J. (2012) identified 4 ways to support new communication partners: -

1: Focus on the learner's skills and communication partner's behaviour.
2: Select learner and communication partner's skills.
3: Practice communication partner skills prior to interactions with the learner.
4: So that the communication partner does not become overwhelmed, begin with small steps to then expand upon and generalise skills.

Importance of Communication Partners

Communication partners and their attitudes and beliefs play an important role in supporting the learners with Speech, Language and Communication Needs (SLCN), and successful use of their AAC system. All communication partners must presume competence and have the belief that all learners have the ability and right to communicate (Biklen and Burke, 2006).

Important Characteristics for Supporting the Learner with Speech, Language and Communication Needs?

The most effective communication partners focus on positive interactions with the learner. They show they value the learner's AAC system and attempts to communicate. Communication partners will comment and add meaning to a learner's message in a supportive environment.

Learners with typically developing speech are immersed in an environment rich in spoken language and will thus develop spoken language. By the time a typically developing child has begun to speak at the age of 18 months they have been exposed to a staggering 4,380 hours of spoken language, without any expectation for the child to communicate using spoken language. Although the child is unable to speak yet, the communication partner uses spoken language with the child from birth.

For a learner who uses aided language/AAC, it is important for the communication partner to use aided language with them. Learners receiving purely spoken language, with no aided language input, will not be able to independently begin using aided language. In order for a learner to become confident and able to effectively use aided language, it is essential the communication partner uses aided language too.

Imagine going on holiday to another country where you do not know the language, as much as you hear the language and are immersed in an environment where everyone is speaking the language, you do not pick up the language yourself. You are unable to understand what is being said around you.

This can be likened to Figure 12.2 of an aided language user.

Now, the person you are talking to begins to use pictures with you. You are able to use these pictures with the person you are communicating with. How much easier would it be to communicate with the person when you have a shared language you can communicate using?

This is shown in this illustration. In Figure 12.3.

Communication Access UK (an initiative led by the Royal College of Speech and Language therapists in partnership with charities, resulting in accreditation to help people living with a communication disability), which can be found here https://communication-access.co.uk/ identified four key elements of success for supporting learners with SLCN, who use aided language/AAC. This includes:

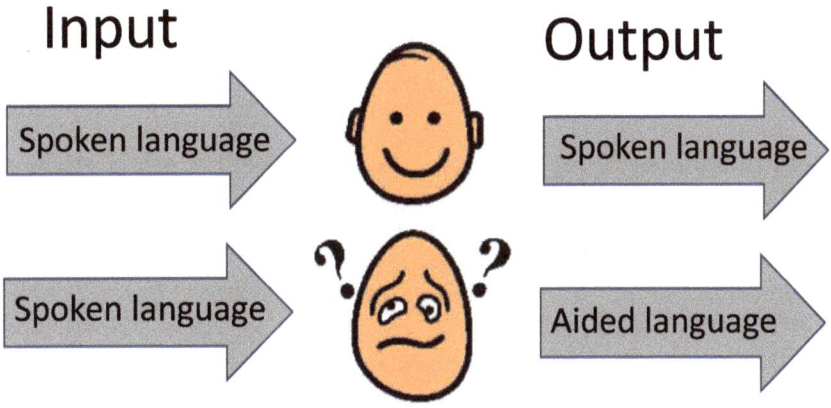

Figure 12.2 Image of 2 faces, with arrows pointing to the right showing spoken and aided language.
Source: Adapted from Porter (2004).

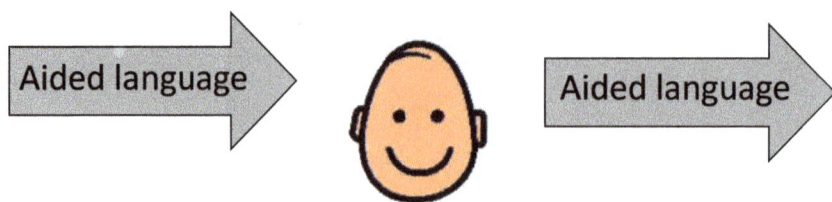

Figure 12.3 Image of a smiling face with arrows pointing to the right showing aided language.

Source: Adapted from Porter (2004).

- *TIME*: when communicating with an individual who uses aided language it will take longer than spoken language. It is important to allow extra time when communicating with the individual.
- *ASK*: when communicating with an individual who uses aided language, ask what helps. It is important to recognise the specific support needs of an individual, for example by simplifying speech, speaking clearly, or providing written support for the individual.
- *LISTEN*: when communicating with the learner who uses aided language, listen and check you have understood what they are communicating, and they have also understood.
- *KEEP TRYING*: when working with an individual who uses aided language, keep trying and learn from mistakes.

Communication Breakdowns

Kent-Walsh and McNaughton (2005) identified the success of communicative interaction as being dependent on the communication skills of each individual communication partner participating in the exchange. In the case of an interaction involving a learner who uses aided language/AAC, the success of the interaction depends not only on the skills of the learner themselves, but also on those of the communication partner.

Communication partners require several characteristics to successfully support a learner with SLCN. Higginbotham, Kim and Scally (2007) identified these as 'interaction characteristics'. They identified the difficulties in initiating and maintaining turn taking in conversations and the need for collaborative message production, and co-construction, between the communication partner and learner using aided language. They identified the barrier of slow production rate of messages (5–15 words per minute) for those learners using aided language/AAC, with frequent misunderstandings and the need for message repairs. They also noted difficulties with the learner initiating conversations with the communication partner.

Lund, S. and Light, J. (2007) identified how discourse, or communication breakdowns, occur when:

- Turn-taking patterns are not equal.
- The communication partner is dominant, for example, takes up twice as many turns; controls the focus of the interaction; and initiates more than half of the topics introduced.
- The learner who uses aided language/AAC has a respondent role, seldom initiating conversation.

Kent-Walsh and McNaughton, (2005, p. 195–204) further identified how discourse, or communication breakdowns occur when:

- Interactions involve questions and answers.
- The communication partner requests yes/no or asks the learner' Who questions (e.g., Who? What? When? Where? Why? How?).

The impact of this on the learner is shown in this table.

Communication partner	Learner using aided language/AAC	Strategies to try
More dominant in conversations	More passive in conversations Does not have control of interactions	Give learners time and space to respond and actively engage in conversation. Draw the learner in and pick up their non-verbal communication.
Take more turns	Take less turns	Engage naturally in a 'my turn, your turn' conversation as you would in everyday conversations. Or simple turn-taking games such as Pop up Pirate.
Ask too many questions	Uses less communicative functions Feels put under pressure	Use the strategy of using 4 statements to every one question, rather than firing questions at the learner expecting a response.
Initiates more frequently	Rarely initiates conversations Have a respondent role	Respond to what the learner has said and provide the learner with a means to initiate conversation and draw attention to themselves without feeling vulnerable and exposed.

In addition to this, if the communication partner has limited skills, knowledge and support regarding aided language and AAC, this can cause communication breakdowns and ultimately AAC system abandonment, especially during periods of transition.

Communication breakdowns can also occur due to the physical limitations of the learner, the relationship the learner has with the communication partner and the AAC system being used. If this is too complex for the learner and challenging for the learner to access, they are more likely to become disengaged and reluctant to communicate using their AAC system (Higginbotham, Kim and Scally, 2007) .

Discussion Point!

- Consider learners within your classroom.
- Have they ever experienced communication breakdowns? What does this look like for them?
- Looking at the reasons for communication breakdowns discussed above, what do you feel was contributing to this breakdown?
- How do you think you could have repaired the communication breakdown?
- What strategies would you put in place to support that learner now?

Level of Prompting a Communication Partner can offer the Learner Who uses Aided Language/AAC

When supporting learners who use aided language/AAC, it is important not to over prompt, allowing time for the learner to respond. This table is an adaption to Rachel Langley's prompt hierarchy, 2015.

1.	Expectant pause	Give the learner the time and opportunity to respond.	
2.	Indirect non-verbal prompt	Use body language to show the learner you are expecting them to do something	• Expectant facial expression • Questioning hand motion • Shrug
3.	Indirect verbal prompt	Use open-ended questions, indicating that you are expecting the learner to do something, without being specific	• Now what? • What should we do next?
4.	Request a response	Direct the child specifically	• Tell me what you want • You need to ask me
5.	Gestural Cue	Use body language to give the learner a specific direction	• Point to the symbol, leave/tap your finger for several seconds to get the learner started with their message
6.	Partial verbal prompt	Give the learner part of the expected answer	• You went to the… • He felt…
7.	Direct model	Model on the learner's AAC system. Pause and wait for the learner to imitate or respond	• You went to the shops • He felt sad
8.	Physical assistant	Use hand over hand support to assist the learner in forming the message on their AAC system	

Copyright material from Katy Leckenby and Meaghan Ebbage-Taylor (2025), *AAC and Aided Language in the Classroom* Routledge

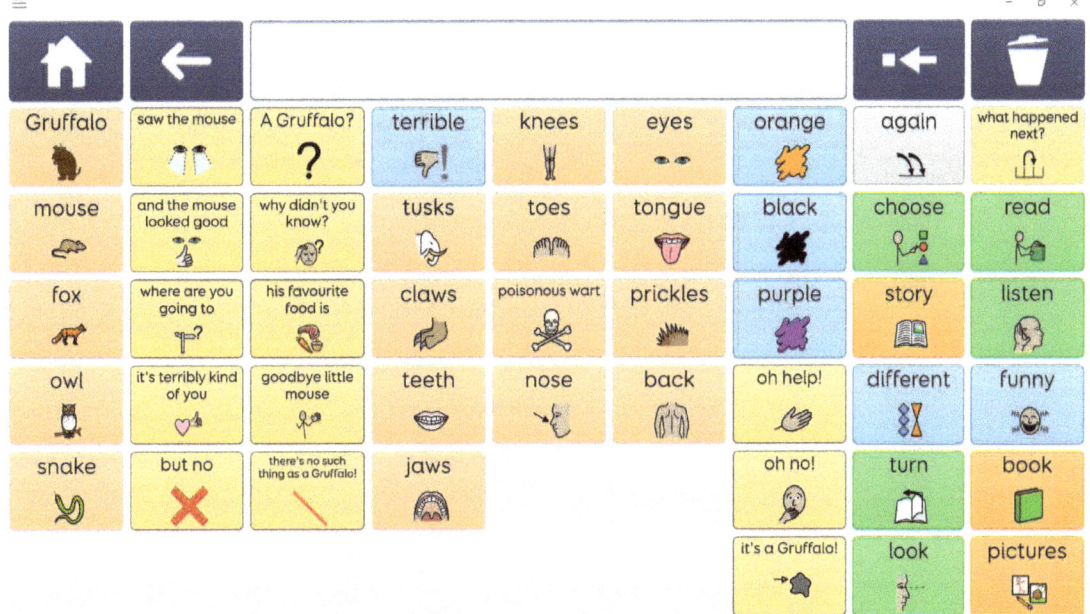

Figure 12.4 This image shows a grid with words relating to Gruffalo.

Source: Smartbox, creators of Grid AAC software.

One example of the use of the prompt hierarchy used in practice is seen below whilst reading *The Gruffalo*. During this activity the communication partner (the teacher) was working with the learner to discuss the conversation between the fox and mouse during the story, using the SuperCore vocabulary (Figure 12.4).

1. The teacher turned the book to this page and awaited a response from the learner.
2. The teacher pulled a scared face, taking a deep breath.
3. The teacher remarked, in a scared voice, 'What is going to happen next?'
4. The teacher proceeded to request a response, 'Can you tell me what's going to happen next?' (this was kept open-ended with several possible answers within the page, for example, 'fox saw mouse' 'oh help!', 'The mouse looked good!', 'His favourite food is fox' and so forth.
5. The teacher pointed to fox on the page and held a finger there to draw attention and focus towards the device.
6. The teacher began the sentence for the learner, 'The fox …' (expecting the ending 'saw the mouse', however this was still kept open-ended, for example the learner could have responded with alternative endings.
7. The teacher modelled for the learner; 'The fox saw the mouse' and left a pause for the learner to respond.
8. The teacher used hand under hand support to create the sentence, 'The fox saw the mouse'.

This prompt hierarchy has since been re-visited by Rachel Langley (2023) (Figure 12.5).

Langley identifies 'healthy habits. These are strategies which are considered both respectful and helpful in teaching autonomous communication. This teaches the learner that using aided language/AAC is a tool to support their communication and they have freedom and autonomy regarding what they want to say and when they want to say it. There is no expectation they will join in and they are able to choose not to participate. These strategies are reflective of those seen in typical language development for learners using spoken language.

1. She describes this as a 'thoughtful' pause rather than an 'expectant' pause, shifting the function of this pause to not put pressure on the learner, inviting rather than expecting them to participate in the activity.
2. Rather than the communication partner using body language to show the learner they are expected to respond, instead the communication partner uses their body language to express interest in the learner, to show they are interested in what the learner has to say rather than focussing solely on what you are expecting the learner to do.

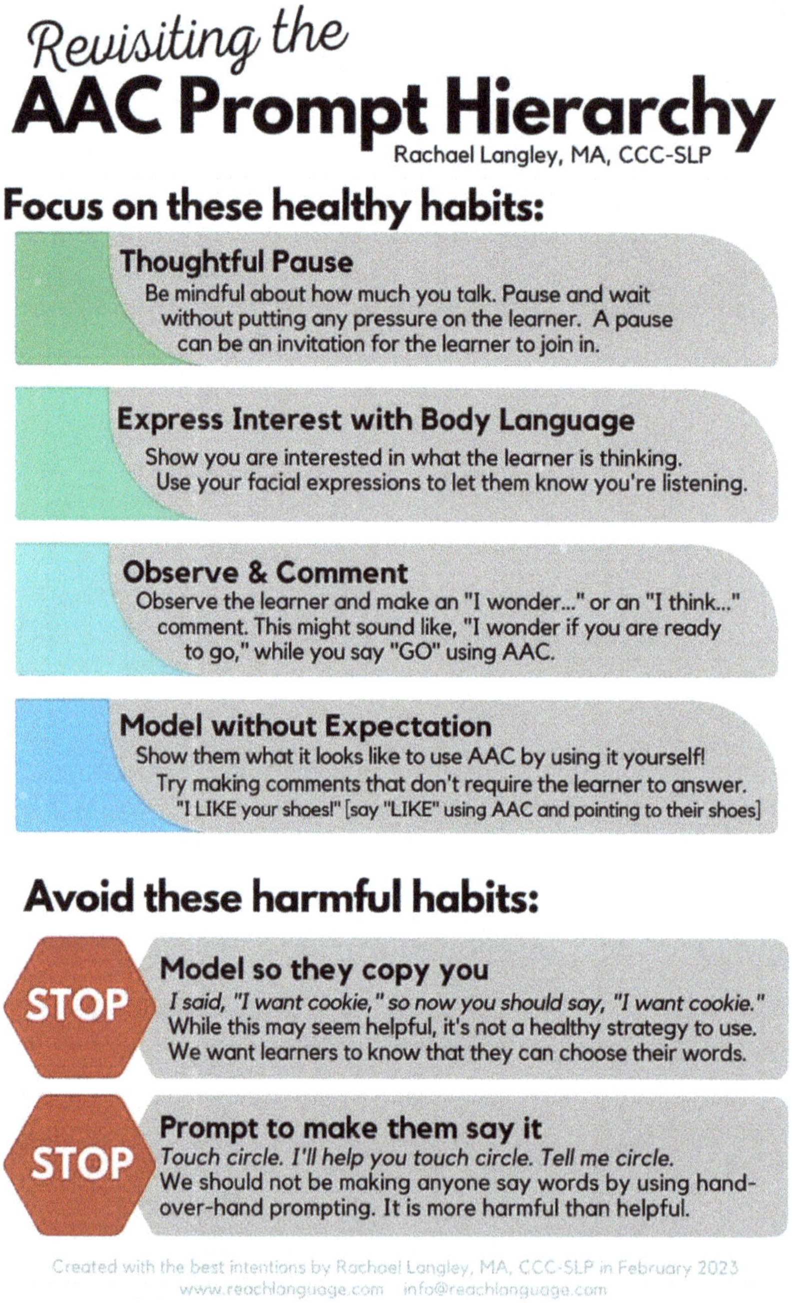

Revisiting the AAC Prompt Hierarchy
Rachael Langley, MA, CCC-SLP

Focus on these healthy habits:

Thoughtful Pause
Be mindful about how much you talk. Pause and wait without putting any pressure on the learner. A pause can be an invitation for the learner to join in.

Express Interest with Body Language
Show you are interested in what the learner is thinking. Use your facial expressions to let them know you're listening.

Observe & Comment
Observe the learner and make an "I wonder..." or an "I think..." comment. This might sound like, "I wonder if you are ready to go," while you say "GO" using AAC.

Model without Expectation
Show them what it looks like to use AAC by using it yourself! Try making comments that don't require the learner to answer. "I LIKE your shoes!" [say "LIKE" using AAC and pointing to their shoes]

Avoid these harmful habits:

STOP — Model so they copy you
I said, "I want cookie," so now you should say, "I want cookie." While this may seem helpful, it's not a healthy strategy to use. We want learners to know that they can choose their words.

STOP — Prompt to make them say it
Touch circle. I'll help you touch circle. Tell me circle. We should not be making anyone say words by using hand-over-hand prompting. It is more harmful than helpful.

Created with the best intentions by Rachael Langley, MA, CCC-SLP in February 2023
www.reachlanguage.com   info@reachlanguage.com

Figure 12.5 This image shows the AAC Prompt Hierarchy'.

Source: Rachael Langley, M.A., CCC-SLP, Speech-Language Pathologist.

3. Observe and comment rather than partial verbal prompting, giving the learner part of the sentence. The communication partner is focussing and observing the learner rather than the activity itself.
4. Model without expectation rather than waiting for the learner to respond. By making these comments that don't require an answer, this takes the pressure off the learner to respond.

It is important that learners have choice over the words they say. Asking the learner to copy a message, this is not a helpful or healthy strategy to use. For example, if the communication partner constructs the message 'I want cookie' and then expects the learner to repeat the same message. This is teaching the learner compliance, rather than autonomy, which will be discussed later in this chapter.

Using hand over hand prompts to make the learner say something, for example 'Touch circle, I'll help you touch the circle, tell me circle' is not giving the learner autonomy over their communication and their actions as they have no control over the communication partner using hand over hand to get them to touch the button on their AAC system for 'circle'.

These habits can stop autonomous communication. In these examples we remove autonomy and take the power of language out of the hands of the learner by asking the learner to say what we tell them to say or direct their hand to point to words and symbols that we as the communication partner have identified as being 'correct'. It is important for the learner to consent to touch, and when we are touching and controlling another person's body, we are in danger of not gaining this consent. Sadly, those with Speech, Language and Communication Needs are often more vulnerable and at risk of abuse, so it is vital we consider carefully using physical prompting and hand over hand support.

Often communication partners with the best intentions can jump straight into the physical support of offering hand over hand support, guiding the learner to the correct vocabulary on a AAC system. This can often be seen in the early stages of The Picture Exchange AAC system, or PECS, however as the learner develops their communication skills and is able to make an exchange independently to aid communication, this is no longer necessary.

Problems with Hand-Over-Hand Prompting

Jane Farrall (2023) discussed the problems associated with hand-over-hand prompting being used as a teaching strategy. This is now viewed as restrictive practice by many communication partners. This is being used within settings without being well informed on the problems surrounding this or developing communication partner's skills to deliver alternative teaching strategies.

Jane Farrall (2023) published the following graphic (Figure 12.6), highlighting the problems with using hand over hand.

Biederman, Fairhall and Davey (1998) demonstrated that passive modelling has a positive impact on learner's progress, calling for a reassessment of current practice and use of hand over hand prompting. Sadly, despite this research being published 25 years ago, little has changed and moved forward in this time and hand over hand prompting continues to be seen in settings.

The use of hand over hand prompting impacts on a learner's autonomy and ability to communicate independently. The learner can then become reliant on this high level of support. It also raises concerns regarding whether we have the right to manipulate and individual's body without consent. This further raises concerns regarding whether we have the right to make someone do what we want, irrespective of whether they want to do it or not and will be made to do it. This causes a power dynamic between the communication partner and learner and causes unease regarding safeguarding relating to the practice of hand over hand. Hand over hand focusses on compliance in contrast to autonomy.

Importance of Autonomy

Autonomy both empowers and motivates learners. Although in society it is important to show compliance when complying to certain rules and expectations, autonomy when communicating is vital. Autonomous communication enables the learner to say whatever they want to say, whenever they want to say and to whoever they want to say it to (Porter, 2018). Autonomy is also important to raise a learner's engagement and self-determination. It gives the learner power and control over their communication. Autonomy also increases an individual's capacity to make decisions and problem solve.

It is important to ensure a balance between autonomy and compliance. Erin Sampson (2021) identified autonomy and compliance being two sides of balancing scales (Figure 12.7).

At times when the learner is showing compliance, the scales become unbalanced, with the learner having less autonomy. This balance alters throughout a learner's day dependent on the task, activity or situation arising. For example, if the fire alarm were to sound, the learner would be required to show compliance by evacuating the building, whereas the learner could have autonomy over what to eat for lunch.

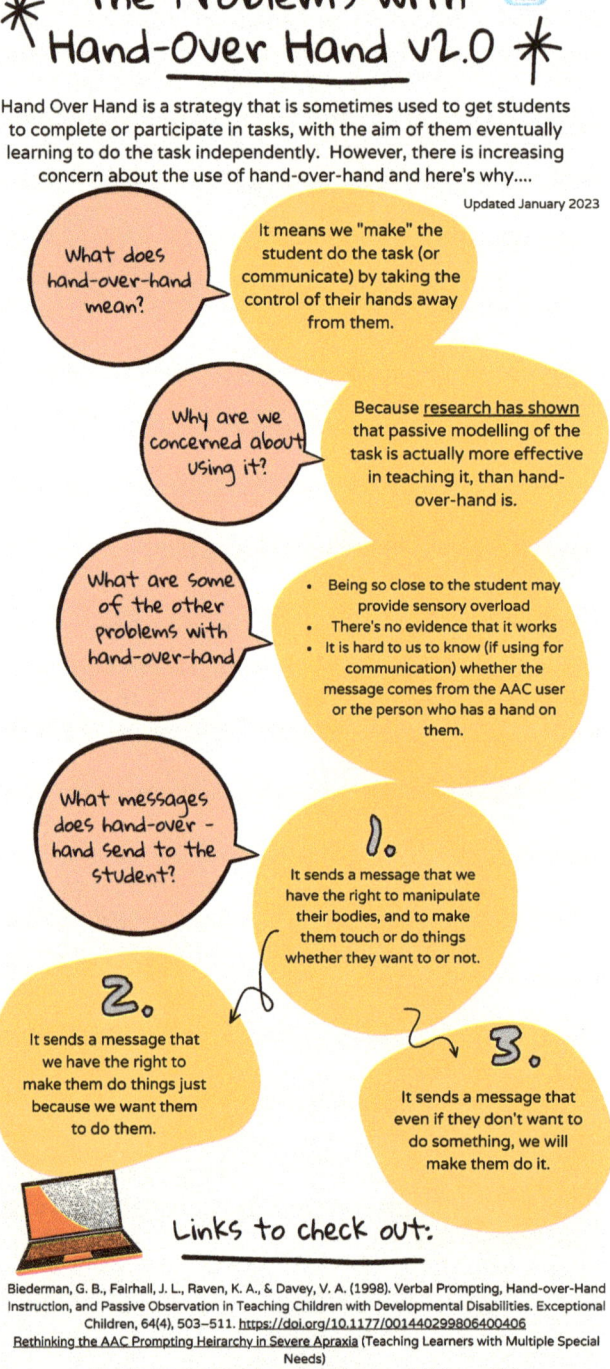

Figure 12.6 This image shows labelled problems with hand over hand.
Source: Jane Farrall of Jane Farrall Consulting. www.janefarrall.com

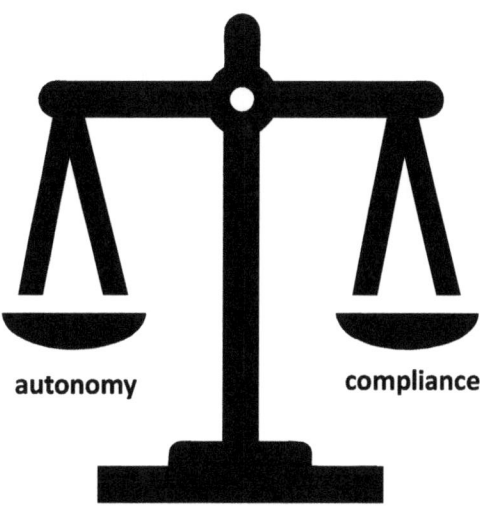

Figure 12.7 An image of weighing scales with autonomy on one side and compliance on the other.

Source: Adapted from Erin Sampson (2021).

When considering the difference between compliance and autonomy, consider these examples.

	Compliance	Autonomy
What do you want for dinner?	Pasta	I don't want dinner! I had too much to eat at lunch!
It's time for swimming.	OK	I'd rather go horse riding than swimming!
Would you like to go to the park?	Yes	I want to go high on the swing!
We're going to read this book.	OK	We read that one yesterday! Can we read this one today?
Do you want the red or blue pen?	Blue	Neither, I want to use the orange one!

Discussion Point!

- Consider times throughout the day when you express autonomy over compliance.
- Can you think of opportunities to enable your learners to express autonomy?
- Can you think of a range of examples you can implement within you classroom practice across the day?
- What impact will this have on your learners?

Directive versus Non-directive Language

It is important for the communication partner to consider the language they use with the learner, using non-directive, rather than directive language. This moves the focus of conversations away from being viewed as testing.

The table below shows examples of non-directive, versus directive teaching (Nervers, 2015).

Directive teaching	Non-directive teaching
Communication partner directs, or expects a specific response from the learner	Communication partner provides input which does not direct the learner to say or do something
Student's response is right or wrong	Communication partner makes comments
Student errors are a possibility	Communication partner makes observations
Communication partner asking questions with a known answer	Communication partner provides the language which may match the learner's experience in the moment

Directive teaching	Non-directive teaching
Communication partner asking test questions to engage the learner	Communication partner models, or shows and 'thinks aloud' where appropriate
Communication partner ignoring learner's communication in favour of more desired formats	Communication partner models use of the learner's AAC system without the expectation that the learner will use it
Directing students to perform	

Example of directive and non-directive teaching include:

Directive Language

This directs the user as to what to say, which explicitly has right and wrong answers. This turns communication into testing. Examples of these include:

- Show me ...
- Point to ...
- Say ...
- Find the ...
- Tell me ...
- Where's the ...
- What do you want? (answer is known)
- What is it time for? (on the schedule)
- Where are we going? (already known)
- Can you find the ...?
- Can you tell me again on your AAC system?

Non-directive Language

Non-directive language does not require a specific response, with no right or wrong answer. This mimics natural conversations, based upon observations, statements and comments. Examples of these include:

- I wonder ...
- I think ...
- I am going to ...
- I see you are ...
- That makes me think ...
- That would make me feel ...

> **Discussion Point!**
>
> - Consider your interactions with learners in your classroom.
> - Observe your learner when communicating with familiar communication partners.
> - Identify what category the interactions fits into:
> - Adult:
>   - Question: asking for information, expecting an answer.
>   - Directive: telling the student what to do/not do.
>   - Statement: comment, give information, no student reply expected.
> - Student
>   - Response: action or message in reply to adult question.
>   - Initiation: spontaneous interaction.
> Collect sample data using the table, creating a tally of interactions.

Communication partner			Learner	
Question	Directive	Statement	Response	Initiation

This chart can help you see the balance of communication turns between the communication partner and learner, and the learner's opportunity to be taught and tested. This will allow you to reflect on your interactions and consider how to focus more on non-directive teaching.

An example conversation and table is completed below:

Communication partner: *Are you ready for play time?*
Learner: *Yes*

Communication partner: *What do you want to do for playtime?*
Learner: *Looks at AAC system and points to ball.*

Communication partner: *Which ball do you want? The big ball or little ball?*
Learner: *Gestures towards the big ball.*

Communication partner: *Find it on you AAC system.*
Learner: *No response*

Communication partner: *Come on, you know where to find it.*
Learner: *No response*

Communication partner: *Let me show you!*
Learner: *Finds big on AAC system with support.*

Communication partner: *That is a big ball!*
Learner: *Says 'big' using AAC system.*
Learner: *Says 'want big' on AAC system.*

Communication partner: *Great, let's play with the big ball.*
Learner: *Says 'like' on AAC system.*

Communication partner: *I like it too.*

When considering questioning, this can be broken down into both open and closed questions. Open-ended questions are less directive than closed questioning.

Open-ended questions have no right or wrong answer, as seen with closed questions. Learners do not feel pressured to give a specific response. They give the learner the opportunity to learn how to communicate how they think and feel and are based upon the learner's own knowledge and feelings. Open-ended questions enable the learner to construct a response based on their own experiences and requires more thought from the learner.

Open-ended questions foster an environment which focuses on rich conversations and meaningful interactions, where the opinion of the learner is heard, and the learner has the confidence to say what they want to say, rather than what they feel they are expected to say. Learners feel their views will be valued and respected, and learners can make decisions for themselves. Ultimately, this builds autonomy to say whatever they want to say, whoever they want to say it to, whenever they want to say it (Porter, 2018).

Communication partner			Learner	
Question	Directive	Statement	Response	Initiation
llll llll	llll llll	ll ll	llll	ll

Figure 12.8 A worked example of a completed communication turns table.

Source: Created by the author.

This example relates to a lesson focussing on reading comprehension.

Closed questions	Open questions
What is the title of the book?	Looking at the title of the book, what do you predict the book may be about?
What is the name of the main character?	Can you describe the main characters?
What is the setting for the story?	What would you do if you visited the setting?
What happened in the beginning of the story?	Why do you think the author decided to begin the book in this way?
How did the character feel?	What do you think could happen to make the character feel differently?
What time of day was it in the story?	Why do you think the story was set at this time of day?

Discussion Point!

Thinking of the Gruffalo example used earlier in this chapter, can you think of some open-ended questions to use?

Means, Reasons and Opportunities

An effective communication partner does not solely provide the learner with their AAC system and a means to communicate, but also generates reasons and opportunities to enable the learner to communicate using aided language/AAC. When these are all in place, the richest communication occurs. This is seen in this diagram (Figure 12.9).

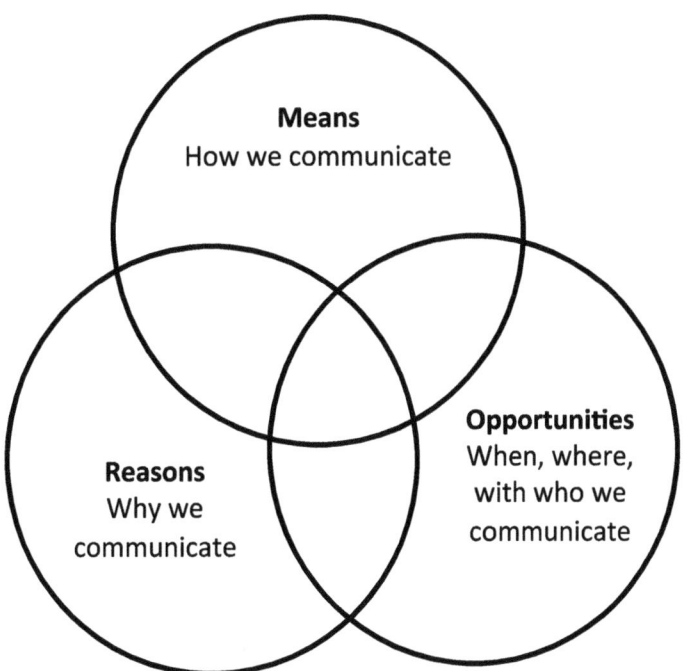

Money and Thurman's model of communication (1994)

Figure 12.9 This image shows 3 circles labelled means, reasons and opportunities.

Source: Created by the author, adapted from Money and Thurman's model of communication (1994).

Examples of these include:

Means (how we communicate)

- Signs
- Symbols
- Gestures
- Body language
- Facial expressions
- Pointing
- Objects and pictures
- Behaviour

Reasons (why we communicate)

- Attention
- Greetings
- Wants/needs
- Request information
- Give information
- Ask questions
- Protest
- Express feelings
- Make choices
- Voice preferences

Opportunities (where, when and with whom we communicate)

- Communication partner
- Time and place
- Shared language
- Shared AAC system
- Shared interests

It's important to ensure there is opportunities throughout a learner's day to use their AAC system in different contexts. This can be created through:

- Routines, which are predictable and repetitive, allowing regular practise of skills.
- Integrating functional activities, which are meaningful and likely to be generalised into a learner's life.
- Avoid tasks which are too cognitively demanding in exchange for activities which are fun, playful, and engaging for the learner.

All communication partners should be considered, but skills will vary across these, with different strategies being used in different environments, for example the difference between home and school.

Sabotage can be a valuable skill for the communication partner to provide the learner opportunities to communicate. The main types include:

- Giving the learner an incorrect item
- Miss out a required item
- Omit a step require to carry out a task
- Not finish a step required to carry out a task

An example of this can be seen below:

Painting a picture:

- Giving the learner an incorrect item – give the learner pencils rather than paints.
- Miss out a required item – give the learner paints, but no paintbrushes.
- Omit a step required to carry out a task – try and paint the picture just stroking the paintbrush on the paints with no water so that they do not pick up any paint.
- Not finish a step required to carry out a task – do not wash the paintbrush between colours, so that they all get mixed together!

Coaching Communication Partners

Coaching unfamiliar communication partners can successfully support learners who use aided language /AAC.

Coaching is a collaborative process involving all parties working together, rather than having an expert. This can lead to communication partners being required to change their habits to use strategies in a specific way to alter their communication with the learner. This can involve direct instruction, practise, evaluation, and peer support. This process is not always easy, so it is important they themselves feel supported. Coaching communication partners will support the establishment of positive interactions with the learner. Then the communication partner acquires the skills to support communication and give effective opportunities, rather than dominating interactions. Coaching can develop communication partner's confidence in encouraging everyone to be encouraged and engage in conversations.

Discussion Point!

- Can you think of opportunities to incorporate sabotage into your day?
- How do you think your learners would react?
- What language could you model with them in these situations?
- Can you use this as a method to practice non-directive teaching?
- What open-ended questions could you ask?

Conclusion

This chapter considered the key role communication partners play in supporting learners who use aided language/AAC. It identified the key skills required to facilitate learner's autonomous communication and offered strategies how this can be achieved.

The next chapter will look into how to support learners when they can not point to symbols on their AAC system or aided language displays.

Bibliography

Biederman, G.B., Fairhall, J.L., Raven, K.A. and Davey, V.A. (1998). Verbal Prompting, Hand-over-Hand Instruction, and Passive Observation in Teaching Children with Developmental Disabilities. *Exceptional Children*, 64(4), pp.503–511.

Biklen, D. and Burke, J. (2006). Presuming Competence. *Equity & Excellence in Education*, 39(2), pp.166–175.

Binger C. and Kent-Walsh, J. (2012). Selecting Skills To Teach Communication Partners: Where Do I Start? *Perspectives of the ASHA Special Interest Groups*, 21(4), pp. 127–135.

Blackstone, S. (1999). Communication Partners. *Augmentative Communication News*, 12(1–2), pp.1–16.

Farrall, J. (2023) *The problems with hand over hand*. Available at: www.janefarrall.com/the-problems-with-hand-over-hand-v2-0/ (Accessed 14 January 2024).

Higginbotham, J., Kim, K. and Scally, C. (2007). The Effect of the Communication Output Method on Augmented Interactio*n. Augmentative and Alternative Communication*, 23, pp.140–153.

Kent-Walsh, J. and McNaughton, D. (2005). Communication Partner Instruction in AAC: Present Practices and Future Directions. *Augmentative and Alternative Communication*, 21, pp.195–204.

Langley, R. (2015). *AAC Prompt Hierachy* Available at: www.pinterest.com/pin/169799848428917357/ (Accessed 14 January 2024)

Langley, R. (2023) *Revisiting the Prompt Hierachy.* [FaceBook] 20 February Available at: www.facebook.com/rachaellangleyaac/posts/revisiting-the-prompt-hierarchy-for-aac-part-2-of-4today-i-want-to-share-with-yo/653433146783339/ (Accessed 14 January 2024).

Lund, S. and Light, J. (2007). Long-term Outcomes for Individuals Who Use Augmentative and Alternative Communication: Part I – What is a "Good" Outcome?. *Augmentative and Alternative Communication*, 22. pp.284–99.

Money, D. and Thurman, S. (1994). Talkabout, a Teaching Course. *Bulletin: Royal College of Speech and Language Therapists*, 504, pp.12–13.

Nervers, M. (2015). *Don't Ask, Don't Tell! Non-Directive Teaching.* Available at: www.angelman.org/wp-content/uploads/2015/11/Dont-Ask-Do-Tell-NonDirective-and-Descriptive-Language-102915.pdf (Accessed 14 January 2024).

Porter, G. (2004). Chatting at school? Proceedings-ISAAC conference, Natal Brazil.

Porter, G. (2018). *Pragmatic organisation dynamic display communication books: Introductory workshop*. Melb: Cerebral Palsy Education Centre.

Sampson, J. (2021). The Autonomy Bucket Challenge https://twowaystreet.com.au/2021/10/09/the-autonomy-bucket-challenge/ (Accessed: 9 May 2024).

13 Supporting Access to Aided Language for Learners with Physical Disabilities

This chapter is for those of you who are working with learners with physical disabilities. These are learners who may have a diagnosis such as cerebral palsy and would find it difficult to easily isolate a finger and successfully select a graphic symbol to communicate. Rest assured that aided language is still a viable option for that population of learners, and even the simple paper-based aided language displays and core boards are accessible to learners with physical disabilities with the correct support in place from the communication partner. In this chapter we look at the different access methods a learner may use to communicate

As technology evolves, so does assistive technology, whether this is using external devices such as eye gaze cameras or accessibility features in mainstream software such as iPhone Operating System (iOS) accessibility features. This chapter will look at some of the current access methods and considerations around using these access methods for communication.

When a child has a physical disability and access methods have to be considered, there should be an understanding that learning an access method is one skill and developing language skills using aided language is another skill. There is an expectation for the learner to learn skills in two different areas before they can have success in using that access method to effectively communicate with the aided language. Educators are expecting the combination of language development and access skills to be at a competent level. Often without direct instruction in either area on language acquisition or access skill development. Figure 13.1 clearly highlights the demands we are placing on learners when they are using a new access method.

If you are unsure of what access method might be most appropriate for your learner, there is a helpful guidance questionnaire that can help to steer you in your journey. It is called the Universal Core Selection Tool, and it was created by the Center for Literacy and Disability Studies at The University of North Carolina, as part of their Project Core Implementation Model, which was aimed at supporting educators to implement the use of core language in educational settings. It has questions such as:

- Does the student have any useful vision?
- Is the student able to physically point?
- Can the student learn to reliably use eye gaze to make a selection?

Touch Access

Skill Development

Touch access is often seen as self-explanatory and is often overlooked when we think of adaptations or skill development that is needed for success. Touch access is classed as direct access.

When thinking about touch access to paper-based resources, there are ways that we can facilitate more effective access by how we present the paper-based resources to the learner. Figure 13.2 is an example of a core word board which could be accessed by a learner who is unable to isolate a finger but is able to fist point.

When thinking about using electronic AAC it may be worthwhile to consider how touch screen devices evolved over the years. Initially, touch screens just required the user to tap or press the screen, then in 2007 came the first smart phone, the iPhone, and suddenly how we interacted with touch screens began to change. If you think about how you interact with your smart phone, you will realise that how you touch the screen varies on the task you are trying to accomplish. You may swipe the screen, you may press a target on the screen, you may pinch and drag out to enlarge something on the screen or you might press and hold an area to select something.

DOI: 10.4324/9781003410836-13

Consider the complexity and identify activity/task, communication system/cognition and physical access as **RED, YELLOW** or **GREEN**

- Match **RED** cognitive and linguistic tasks with **GREEN** communication systems and positions.

- Match **YELLOW** cognitive and linguistic tasks with **YELLOW** or **GREEN** communication systems and positions.

- Match **GREEN** cognitive and linguistic tasks with **RED** or **YELLOW** communication systems and positions.

- Never pair two **RED**s.

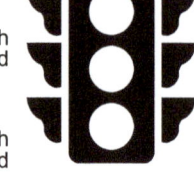

Figure 13.1 Image of a set of traffic lights.

Source: Created by the author.

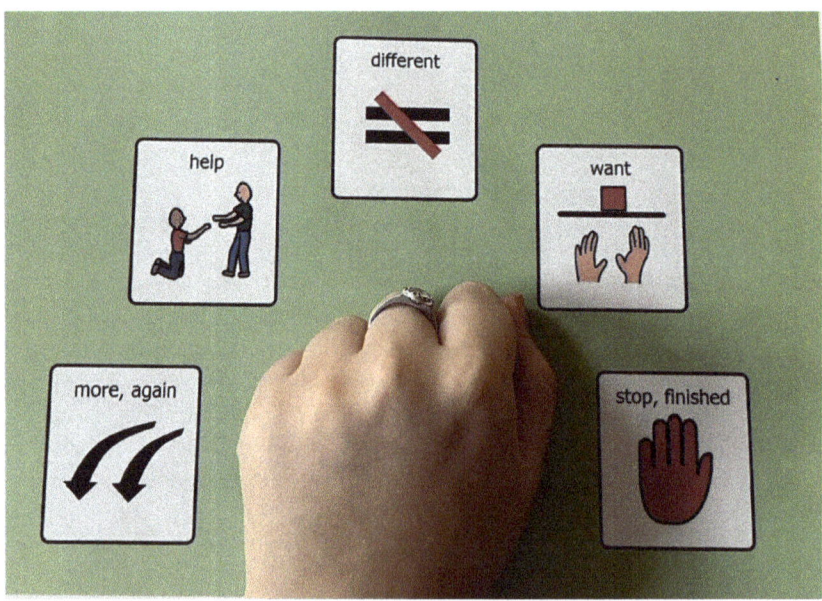

Figure 13.2 Image of a fist on a symbol mat.

Source: Photographed by the author, created by Ace Centre. https://acecentre.org.uk/resources

How you interact with the screen depends on what app you are using. For learners who are using touch access on an electronic communication aid, such as a communication app on an iPad, you need to think about how the learner needs to interact with the app to control it successfully. Some communication apps can use a swipe gesture, but the majority require precise targeting on the screen to make an accurate selection of symbols. Many apps that the learner has experienced previously are apps such as YouTube, which auto generates content from your most commonly watched videos, meaning that when a learner swipes through the videos offered, there is generally a video they find acceptable to watch, making it an error-free activity. Once the learner begins to use a communication app on a touch screen, the task is no longer errorless, which means targeting must be precise. Providing apps with games where targeting has to be precise on the page is a good way to support skill development and also to help you to identify if the learner needs additional support and/or aids to be put in place to better facilitate touch access. Teaching that you need to press specific targets on a touch screen is a necessary skill for most electronic AAC.

Language versus Access

The first consideration should always be how many targets can the learner touch, with accommodations in place, rather than to reduce the amount of language on the aided language

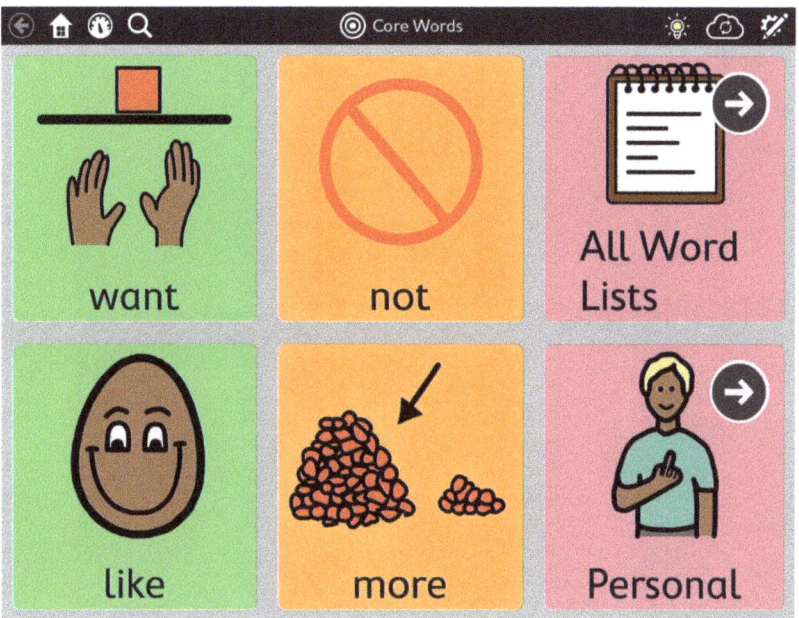

Figure 13.3 Screenshot of a grid of 6 symbols with a green column at the start.

Source: PCS and Boardmaker are trademarks of Tobii Dynavox LLC. All rights reserved. Used with permission.

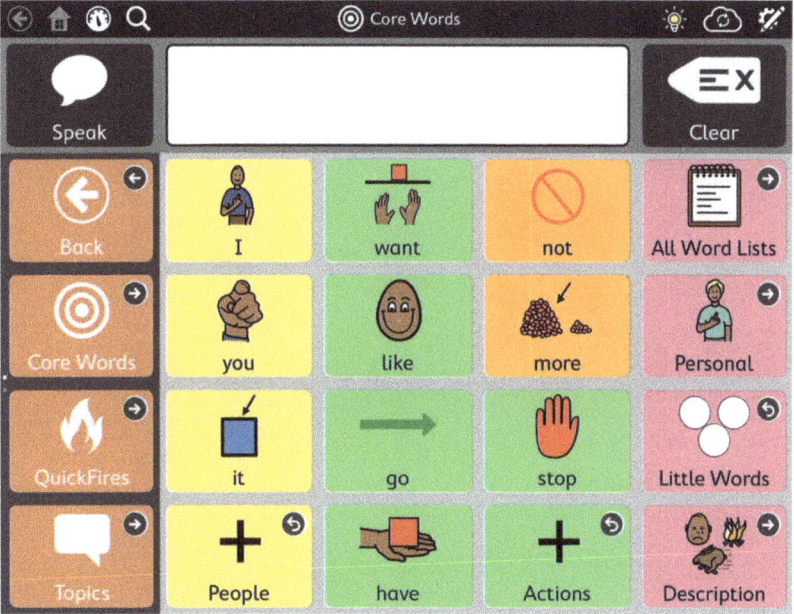

Figure 13.4 Screen shot of grid of symbols with and orange column at the start.

Source: PCS and Boardmaker are trademarks of Tobii Dynavox LLC. All rights reserved. Used with permission.

display/AAC system to make the targets bigger. Figure 13.3 is an example of the TD Snap Core First vocabulary set at a 2 by 3 grid size. Although these targets may be big enough for the learner to easily touch without making errors, the amount of language they have access to on the page is very limited and therefore could hinder their language development.

If we compare it to a 4 by 4 grid size (Figure 13.4), you can straight away see that the learner has access to a lot more language.

Additional Supports

One way to support touch access is to use aids such as a stylus. Here is a selection of different styli. Ball Stylus Figure 13.5

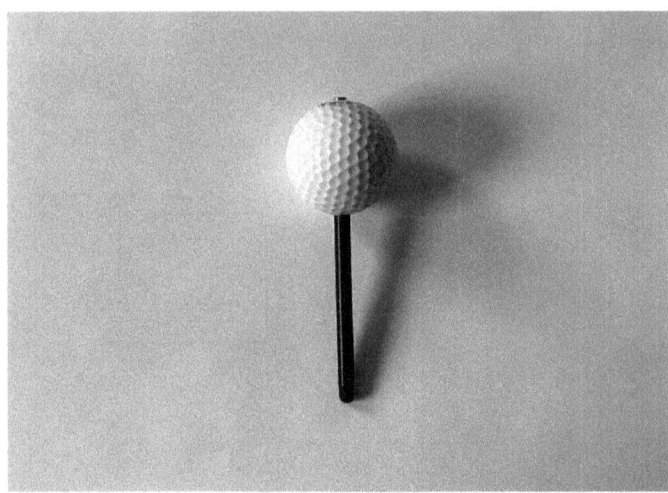

Figure 13.5 Small ball stylus.
Source: Photographed by the author.

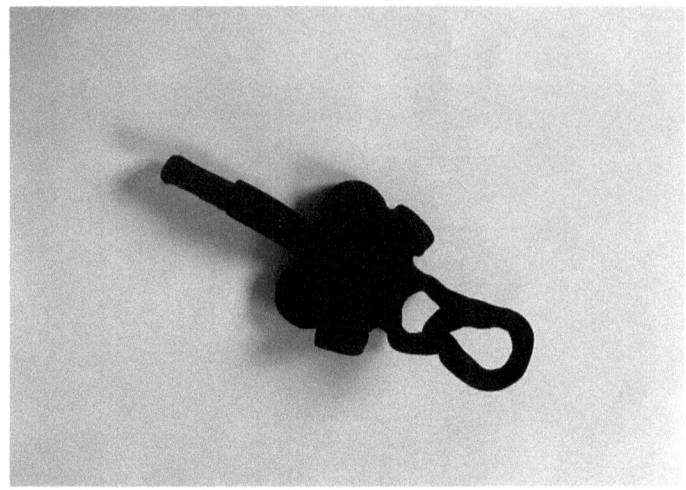

Figure 13.6 Black mouldable stylus.
Source: Photographed by the author.

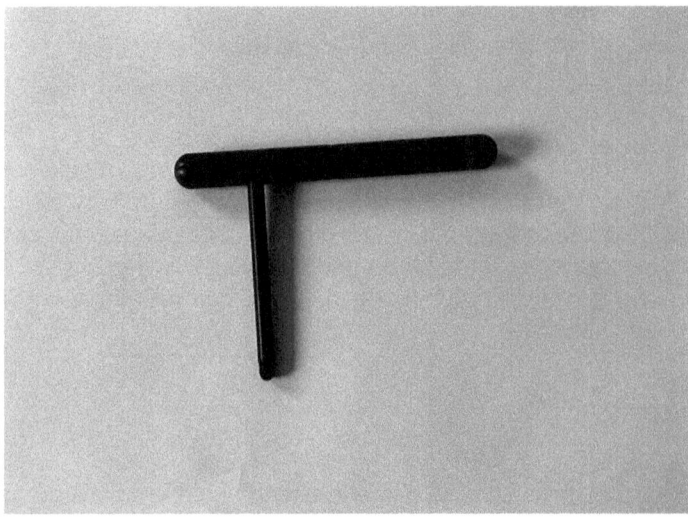

Figure 13.7 Adjustable T-Bar stylus.
Source: Photographed by the author.

Another support can come in the form of Keyguards or Touch Guides. These are designed to support learners who have accidental presses on the screen with other parts of their hands whilst trying to make a selection. Keyguards and Touch Guides can typically be purchased from AAC suppliers, for example, where the electronic communication aid was purchased from. They need to match the learner's specific vocabulary package if they are to be used successfully.

Example of a Keyguard Figure 13.8

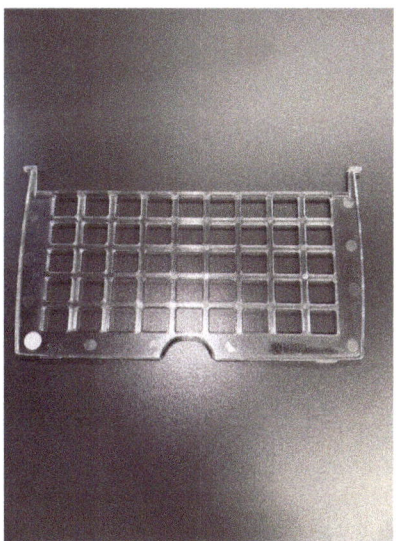

Figure 13.8 Plastic keyguard with rectangular cut outs.

Source: Photographed by the author.

Keyguards sit on top of the touch screen and separate out the targets on the screen into clear sections with the plastic overlay.

Example of a Touch Guide Figure 13.9

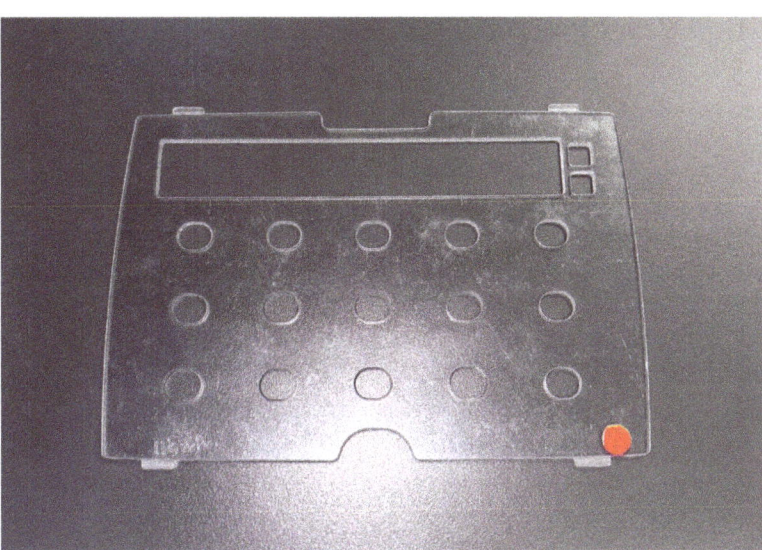

Figure 13.9 Plastic touch guide with circular cut outs.

Source: Photographed by the author.

Touch Guides sit on top of the touch screen and cover the majority of the screen. It has small holes cut out to sit over target areas on the screen, which are designed for the learner's finger tips to be pushed through to trigger the desired target. Touch Guides are useful for learners who may need to rest their hand on the screen. The Touch Guide protects from accidental triggers when a learner does this.

Positioning of the Screen

Another way to support learners is to think about the positioning of the touch screen. Some learners may benefit from the screen being at arm's length away because when their arms lock in extension, they find it easier to then be stable to target an area on the screen with their fingers. This may mean using items such as table mounts or cases with kick stands to get the angle of the screen in the most efficient place for the learner.

Inbuilt Accessibility Features

Most mainstream software now has accessibility features built in. Most have options around the length of time you have to tap/touch the screen before the selection will trigger, and a feature to ignore repeat presses, for example, when a learner presses the same target twice in quick succession. IOS has additional features, such as initial and final touch, where the first place the learner touches on the screen will be selected. This setting is useful for learners who make a selection and then trail their fingers down the screen afterwards. Turning on initial touch, in touch accommodations, ensures the device doesn't take the trailing hand interaction as a selection, as it will only select the place of initial touch. Likewise, some touch screen users will travel across the screen to land on the target they wish to select, before removing their hands from the screen. For those learners the IOS setting of Final Touch in Touch Accommodations would be more beneficial. Accessibility settings within mainstream software is constantly evolving, so it is always worthwhile considering how your learner is interacting with the touch screen and looking at interaction settings within the accessibility settings.

Scanning

This can be split into two distinct methods of scanning, which require similar skills from the learner, one with the use of Assistive Technology, and one without. These two methods are called Partner Assisted Scanning and Switch Scanning/Switch Access.

Partner Assisted Scanning

This is where the communication partner reads out the symbol options/choices available, in a list style and the learner indicates a yes response when the communication partner gets to the option the learner wants to select and speak. An example of this may be a communication partner pointing to symbol options on an aided language display and then saying the symbol selected when the learner indicates a 'yes' response.

If you were supporting a learner with this core board (Figure 13.10), you would say: like, want, not, go, and when the learner indicated their yes response, you would verbally say the word they selected, for example, 'go'. Then you might respond 'Oh, you want to go now' or apply it to the context you are in. Maybe it is close to home time, and you may say 'Oh, do you want to go home?'

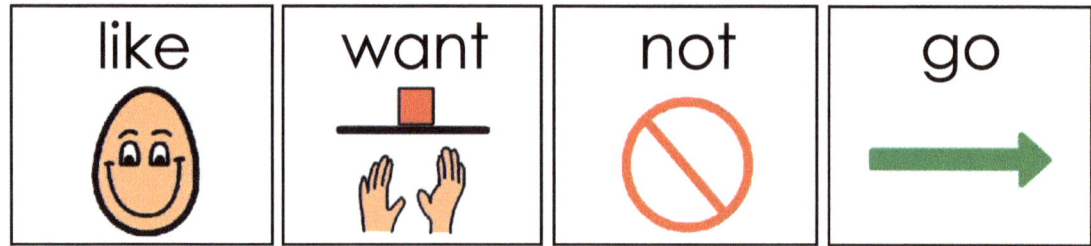

Figure 13.10 A row of four symbols beginning with like.

Source: University of North Carolina at Chapel Hill, The Center for Literacy and Disability Studies, www.project-core.com.

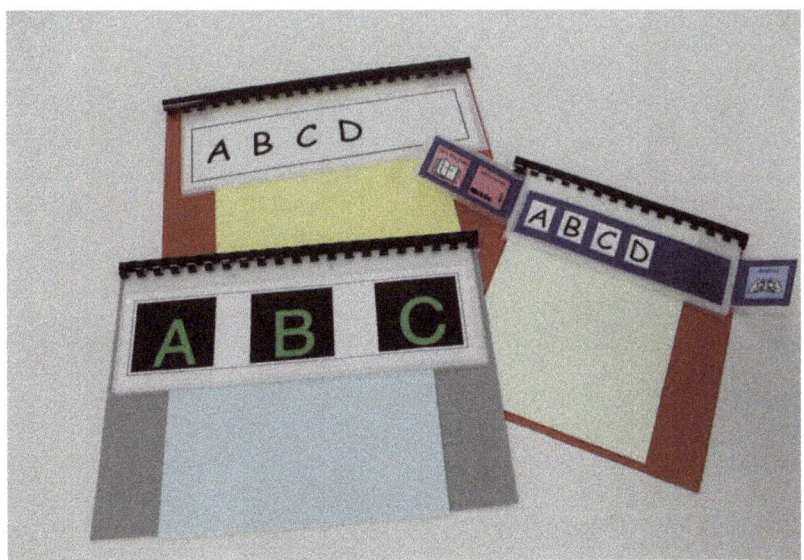

Figure 13.11 Three folders displaying letters.

Source: Photographed by the author.

Likewise, this could be done with the letters of the alphabet with a learner who is developing their writing skills with an alternative pencil. Remember, a child who first picks up a pencil can't write their name. They begin by exploring the writing tool, they scribble, and mark make. Children with complex physical disabilities also need the opportunity to explore a writing tool. Figure 13.11 is an image of an alternative pencil which the learner can access with partner assisted scanning.

The bonus of partner assisted scanning instead of switch scanning on an electronic AAC device, is that you can see the context that is happening around the learner and are therefore more likely to be able to accurately interpret the aided language they select. You are also in the position to be able to slow down your speed when reading the selections and waiting for them to refocus if something has just distracted them in the classroom whilst they were communicating with you.

> **Discussion Point!**
>
> Have you ever tried partner assisted scanning with a learner? If not, it might be helpful to grab a friend and have a practice. Practicing away from the live classroom environment can feel less daunting. If you need to see it in practice, there are plenty of example videos on YouTube.

Switch Scanning

A switch is a specialised input device which can enable individuals with limited motor skills or physical disabilities to interact with and control their AAC device. Switches should be considered for learners who cannot use traditional touchscreens, keyboards, or other input methods.

Switches vary in terms of:

Physical Characteristics

- Size and Shape: Switches come in various sizes and shapes to accommodate different user needs. They can range from small buttons to larger, more accessible switches.
- Colour and Design: The switches often have high-contrast colours and clear labels to aid visibility and recognition.

Functionality

- Activation Mechanism: Switches are designed to be easy to press or activate using various body parts or movements, such as a finger, hand, foot, head, or even a puff of air.
- Feedback: Depending on the model, some switches provide tactile or auditory feedback when activated, helping the learner know that their action has been registered on the AAC device.

How they Connect

- Wired or Wireless: Switches can be wired or wireless, depending on the learner's requirements and the AAC system they are using. Some learners prefer not to have wired switches as they get their limbs tangled in the wire. Often schools prefer wired switches as opposed to Bluetooth ones as staff do not have to remember to charge the wired switches, which are simple plug-and-play technology.

Below are examples of some switches and a description of their main features:

Wired Switches

Access Wobble Switch: Figure 13.12: is Switch which uses a wired connection. This is a good switch for a learner who has gross motor movements and needs the switch to move with them, so they don't injure themselves when triggering it. This switch has a spring pole allowing movement when triggered. This switch also gives clear audio feedback via a click when it has been triggered.

Jelly Bean Switch: Figure 13.13: Robust 6.5cm surface area switch. It has a wired connection and gives clear audio feedback in the form of a click when pressed. It is suitable for learner's who need the feedback to know that they have successfully pressed it and also for learners who might apply a lot of force when pressing the switch.

Smoothie Switch: Switch shown in Figure 13.14: Switch has smoothed edges which allows a learner to be able to trigger the switch if they touch the edges, as well as the top of it. Smoothie switches are useful for learners who roll onto switches by rotating their fist.

Pal Pad Switches: The switches shown in Figure 13.15: Flat light touch switches which give no feedback from the switch itself. These switches are designed for learners who have very light

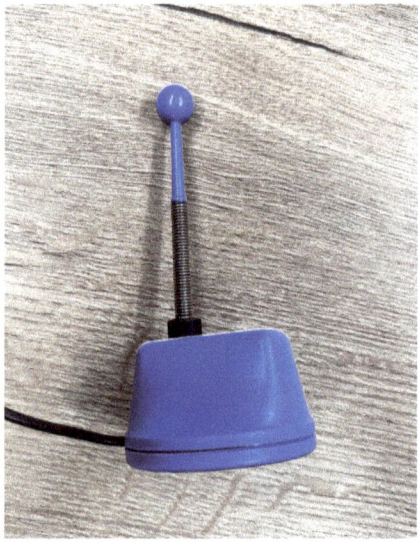

Figure 13.12 A blue switch with a spring with a ball on top.

Source: Photographed by the author.

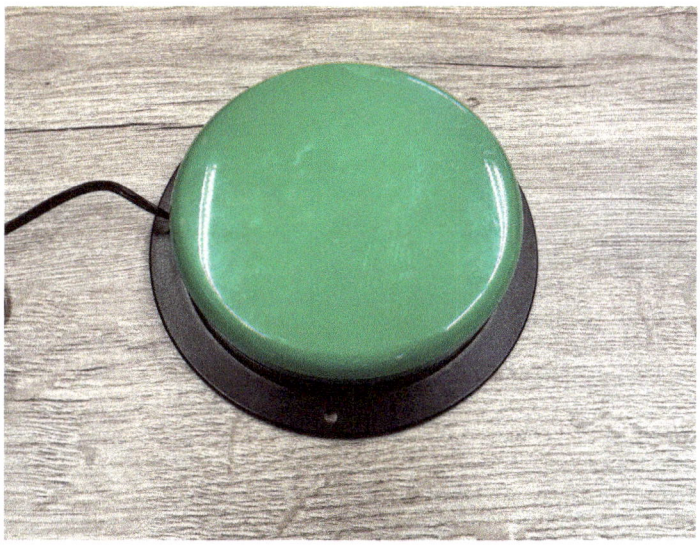

Figure 13.13 A green circular switch.
Source: Photographed by the author.

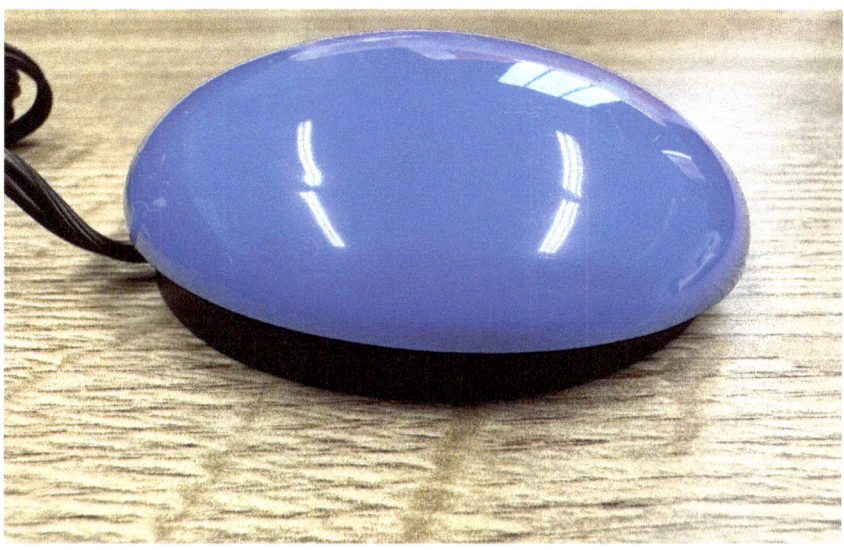

Figure 13.14 A curved edge blue circular switch.
Source: Photographed by the author.

touch or who get too focused on the feedback the switch can offer, rather than the selection/action activated. They come in a variety of sizes.

Pillow Switch: Figure 13.16: Cushioned switch that a learner would typically press with their head to use. The surface is cushioned to ensure that the learner does not experience discomfort when triggering it. They are often attached to the headrest on a learner's wheelchair.

Bluetooth Switches

Blue2 Switch: Bluetooth unit with two switches on the top. It also has two switch ports so other switches can be plugged into it and remain connected via the Blue2 to the device.

iSwitch: Figure 13.17: Bluetooth switch which Includes 24 pre-programmed functions. This allows the learner to input the switch press as different functions on the communication device, for example, space or enter.

This is a very small number of the switches currently available to support learners who would benefit from using switch scanning as an access method. The selection chosen comprise some

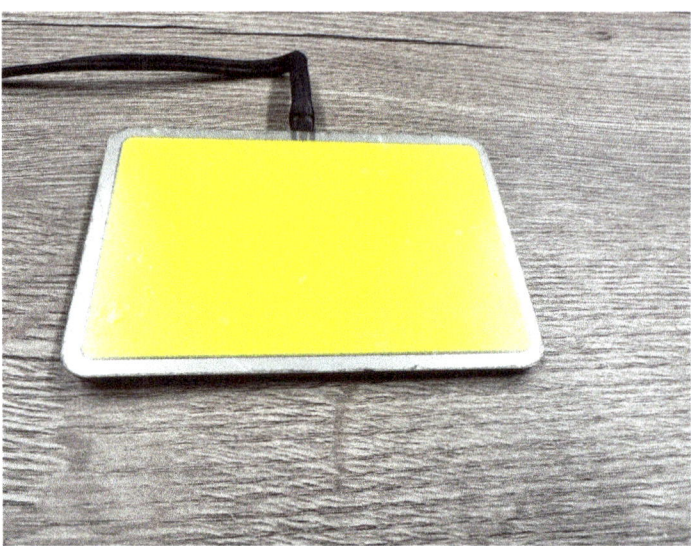

Figure 13.15 A flat, yellow, rectangular switch.

Source: Photographed by the author.

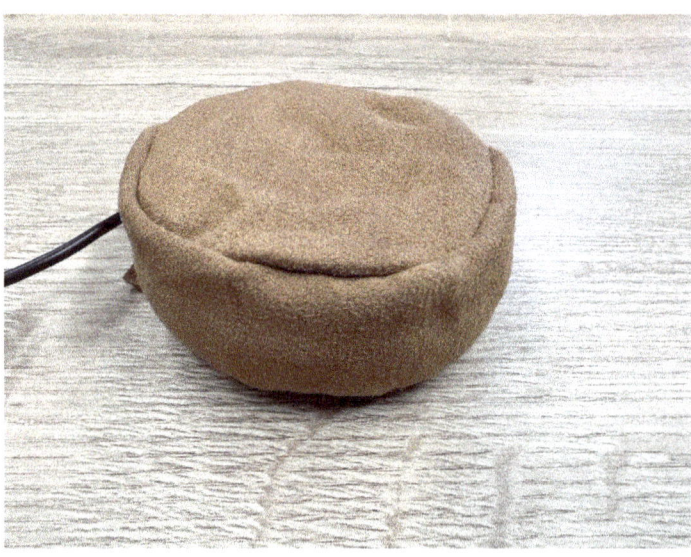

Figure 13.16 A brown, round, fabric switch.

Source: Photographed by the author.

of the switches you may come across – which are more frequently seen in specialist school settings.

When considering switch access, it is advisable to work as part of a multidisciplinary team with the learner's occupational therapist to identify suitable body parts and movement patterns for the learner to trigger the switch or switches, depending on how many suitable control sites the learner has for the switches.

Switch Skill Development

Once the learner is able to physically trigger the switch, they need to develop skills in using the switch to control what happens on the screen of a device. As mentioned at the start of the chapter, learning the skills for the access method – in this case switch skill development – should be done in fun activities with low cognitive demand. It is hard enough learning how to use the switch to control what's on the screen, let alone the task on the device itself also being cognitively challenging. Therefore, developing switch skills is best practiced with highly motivating,

Access to Aided Language for Learners with Physical Disabilities 147

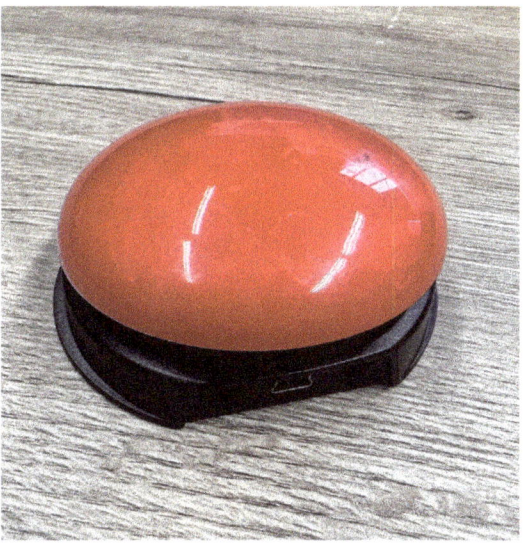

Figure 13.17 A red smooth-edged switch with a chunky black base.

Source: Photographed by the author.

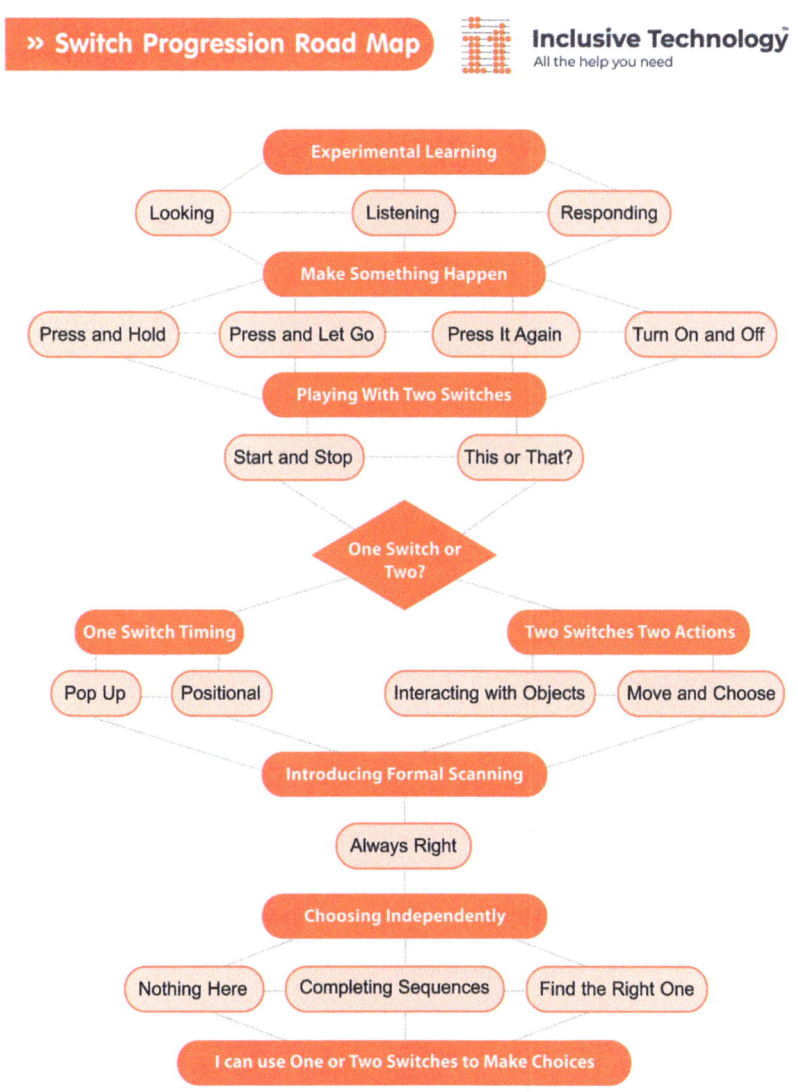

Figure 13.18 A red flowchart.

Source: Switch Progression Road Map, created by Inclusive Technology (2011).

easy activities, such as playing simple games, rather than expecting a learner to be able to jump straight in and control an AAC system with the switch/switches.

There are several supports around the theory of switch-skill development. Each theory suggests a progression through skill levels.

Next is the Switch Progression Road Map, created by Inclusive Technology (2011) based on Ian Bean's theory of switch skill development (Figure 13.18). This documents the range of skills required and the variations educators must consider when supporting a switch user, such as: Would the learner benefit from using one or two switches, depending on whether the learner has two control sites from which they can easily control a switch per site.

Next are the Stepping Stones to Switch Access (Burkhart, 2018).

Stepping Stones to Switch Access

1. Single Switch: Cause-and-Effect
   At this beginning step, the individual begins to associate an intentional movement with the ability to cause something to happen using a switch. Human beings do not learn cause and effect through specific prompting and direct teaching. Individuals learn cause and effect through experiencing the effects of their own random movements via trial and error and then making the connection that they can use one of their current movements to make something happen again. Cause and effect is not a cognitively challenging skill. Children as young as 2 to 3 months demonstrate this skill (Goodwyn, Acredolo, & Brown, 2000). Individuals who have severe physical and multiple challenges may have experienced many random cause-and-effect situations and not had the opportunities needed to naturally develop discrimination of movements and causal relationships. In addition, they may develop learned helplessness and not see themselves as active participants but, rather, as passive beings where things happen to them without their control. For example, it is not uncommon for individuals with severe challenges to learn that switch access is done by waiting for someone to take their hand and activate the switch, with no thought to initiate that movement themselves. It is, therefore, the intent of this stepping stone to engineer experiences that enable the natural process of learning cause and effect to take place through active learning. For many individuals, this step, if done correctly, may only take a few minutes before the learner gets the needed "ah ha" and can move on to the next step. In this author's experience, people learn cause-and-effect very quickly when components are carefully designed. If within three different sessions the individual is not grasping the concept, then each of the many factors (position, movement, switch placement, choice of effect, motivation, relevance, emotional state, and so forth) should be revisited and readjusted as needed.

2. Single Switch: Multiple Locations and Functions
   At this step, the individual understands the most basic concept of cause-and-effect and can now use that knowledge to learn new movements. At this step, the individual needs practice intending and executing movement(s) for different purposes or with different body parts or when a switch is moved to a new location or used for a new function.

3. Two Switches: Two Functions
   Once the individual can access switches in multiple locations for multiple functions, keep motivation and engagement high by using two switches. Automaticity of switch access is not necessary to move to this step. The individual will continue to practice toward developing automaticity using these activities. This step encourages more active cognitive engagement and the development of discrimination and problem solving. Up to this point, the individual's options consisted of 'do it' or 'do not'. Now, two options with different functions are added.

4. Learning to Two-Switch Step Scan
   Some individuals understand the concept of two-switch step scanning and just need more practice. Those individuals may skip this step and move directly to Stepping Stone 5. This step helps individuals learn that one switch moves something along a path (mover switch) and the other switch selects the item at the end of that path (selector switch). Activities are specifically designed to move one item along a path or across a screen with repeated activations of the first switch, whereas the second switch is not

active. Once the item reaches the destination, the first switch stops working, and the second switch becomes active to allow for selection of the destination 40 item. Only one switch is active at a time; therefore, the individual receives clear feedback that assists in learning this process. Modelling of the process by partners taking turns with the individual is an effective strategy at this step.

5. Two-Switch Step Scanning: Failure-Free Learning with Feedback

    This stepping stone provides numerous opportunities to practice switch activation with intent, purpose, and variation. All selections result in some type of feedback, and at this point, there are no right or wrong selections, only selections that have different effects. This format allows an individual to use problem-solving strategies and explore opportunities to select from a variety of options. It is also important at this step that each activity has a user-controlled way to end the activity and select a different activity. The learner is presented with a self-controlled "launcher" or "bookshelf" of activities to select from using two switch step scanning.

6. Two Switch Step Scan to a Target – Activities for Increasing Accuracy and Cognitive Engagement

    Before using this step, individuals must have had numerous opportunities to explore activities in a failure-free manner at Stepping Stone 5. Moving to this step too soon puts too much pressure on the individual to select a specific item without having enough experience to learn the motor–cognitive connection of step scanning. Stepping Stone 6 is designed for those individuals who do not naturally move from random selection to intentional selection after many opportunities. Individuals who are able to select items on the basis of desire may skip this step and move on to Stepping Stone 7. Some individuals need more clear opportunities to select an intended target as is the aim here. One switch moves the cursor, highlighter, or partner's indication over an array of null, blank, or nonselectable items. The second switch activates/selects the one active target in the array.

7. Practise for Increasing Accuracy with Two-Step scanning

    At this step, the individual is developing the ability to integrate the motor component of step scanning with the cognitive component of selecting an item for a desired purpose. Many of the same activities in Stepping Stone 5 may be used at this step. However, items in the array will frequently represent a wider variety of desirable and undesirable options. Activities at this level may be failure free with feedback, or they may contain right and wrong options: as long as every option provides clear feedback. At this stage, a simple powerful electronic AAC scanning page set (Cotter, Porter, and Burkhart, 2016) may be introduced along with the individual continuing to use a robust nonelectronic communication system that would require less refined motor skills to access.

8. Switch Automaticity: Reducing time for success and demonstrating Knowledge

    Automaticity of switch access has now been reached, and scanning switch access may be used for more challenging and functional tasks. This level must be reached before scanning may be used as a means for testing knowledge. The individual now has sufficient automaticity with the motor access to the switches to focus on the generation of language and pragmatic discourse for interactive communication. A full robust AAC electronic page set that parallels the individual's nonelectronic AAC system is utilized for communication in a wide variety of contexts. Social and strategic competencies of using electronic AAC may now be further taught and practiced.

In 2020 the Pace Centre created a new support tool called the "Seven Stages of Switch Development" (Figure 13.19). 'The framework provides a helpful reference for measuring and tracking progress while offering flexibility to accommodate the unique needs and preferences of each switch user.'

This tool is freely available, so if you find yourself working with a learner who would benefit from using switch access, this tool will be a helpful resource to guide you both on the journey. The Seven Stages of Switch Development give the learner ownership of their skill development journey and use fun, animated characters to make the tool more user friendly. Pace Centre surveyed educators and established that many felt there was no consistency with work around switch skill progression and that there were no formal means to record a learner's progression. Following this The Pace Centre created a suite of support tools such as: A story book series, information sheets, an assessment tool and training packages.

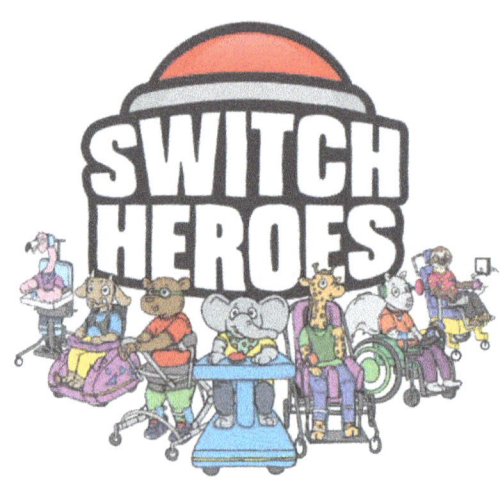

Figure 13.19 Switch Heros logo.

Source: Created by Pace Centre. https://thepacecentre.org/sevenstages/

The characters represent different stages in switch skill development:

Stage 1: Learning by experience - Exploring Egbert
Stage 2: Intentionally make happen - Journeying Jiao
Stage 3: Playing with two switches - making two things happen – Growing Gareth
Stage 4: Using 2 switches for one activity – Budding Brayton
Stage 5: Playing with two switch scanning - Error friendly learning – Flourishing Fatima
Stage 6: using switch scanning - finding the right one – Succeeding Saffi
Stage 7: Independent in functional use – Celebrating Syed

All of these resources are freely available for use at www.thepacecentre.org

Companies such as Inclusive Technology have catalogued interactive games on their website www.HelpKidzLearn.com according to switch skill development, so educators can easily find games appropriate to the learner's switch skill level to support continued switch skill development.

Once a learner has become a proficient switch user, then they can use it as an access method for their electronic AAC. It is possible to teach switch skills on an electronic AAC device, but then you are forcing the learner to do two difficult things at the same time. That is to learn how a switch can control an electronic AAC device and also how they can communicate using the aided language.

When the learner uses a switch to control an electronic AAC device the vocabulary package will move in scan patterns across the aided language in the system, as in Figure 13.20.

The scan patterns can be changed in the settings of the different vocabulary packages. The speed of the scan can be changed, too. If the learner has two switch sites, they can control the movement of the scan with one switch and then select their choice with the second switch.

The example shown is set to scan down the rows first and then once a row is selected, it will scan from left to right cell-by-cell. The learner's multidisciplinary team of speech and language therapist and occupational therapist will be key in supporting you to assess which is the most appropriate scan pattern for the learner to access the aided language displayed in the electronic AAC.

Figure 13.21 and 13.22 is a selection of some of the scan patterns often used in electronic AAC for switch access users:

Vocabulary packages are often arranged slightly differently for AAC users who are using switch access. Higher frequency language is generally placed closer to the top left of the screen to support the learner to access that language quicker, as they do not take as long to reach those words in the scan pattern.

Figure 13.23 is an example of a frequency layout onscreen keyboard for a learner who is using switch scanning as an access method.

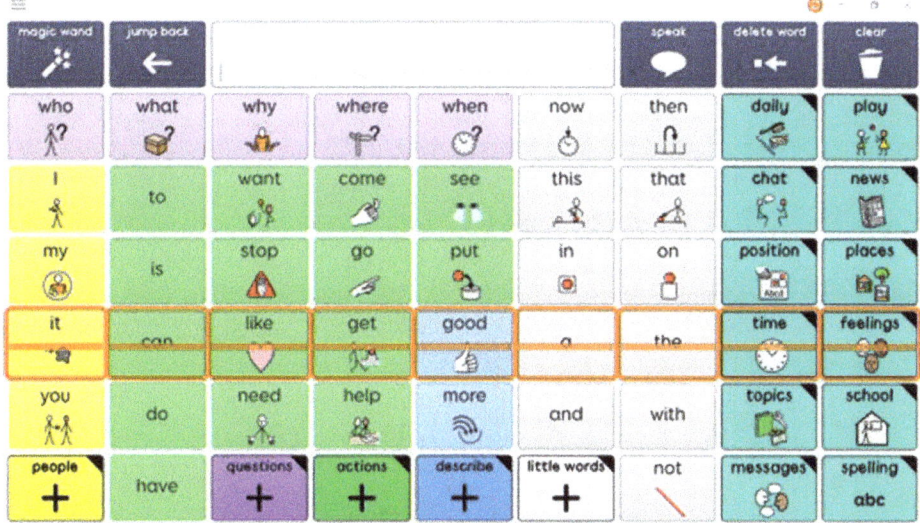

Figure 13.20 Screen shot of grid of symbols with a yellow column at the start. Smartbox, creators of Grid AAC software.

Source: Smartbox, creators of Grid AAC software.

Linear – by indicating each item individually in a consistent linear sequence.

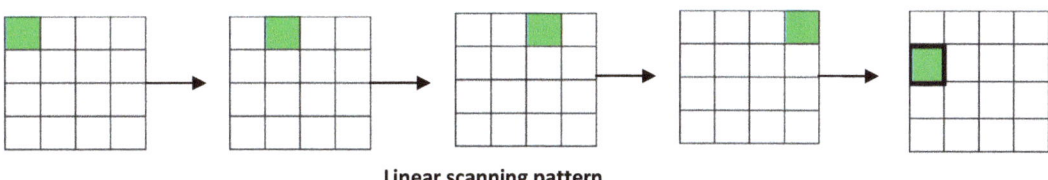

Linear scanning pattern

Row-column or column-row – by indicating each row/column until selected, then scanning each item linearly along the row/column.

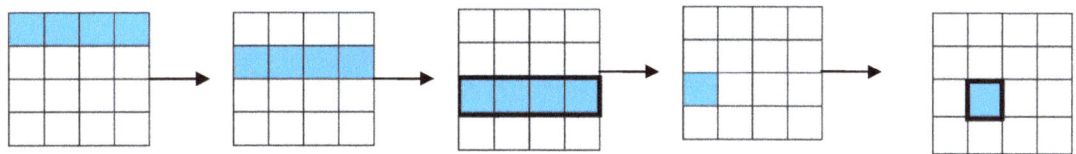

Row/column scanning pattern

Figure 13.21 An image of 10 squares explaining scanning patterns.

Source: Smartbox, creators of Grid AAC software.

Eye Pointing

Eye pointing is where an individual uses their gaze to select symbols, words, or objects on a communication board, computer screen, or other assistive technology device equipped with eye-tracking technology. Eye pointing can be a useful access method to try when other access methods have failed. Eye pointing works by the learner fixating their eyes on specific targets, which the communication partner or computer then reads aloud.

When we think of eye pointing in the classroom environment, most people would jump to the thought of using an eye gaze system to 'unlock' the learner. It is important to remember that eye pointing is an access method, and that there is skill development to be able to use your eyes for communicating, as opposed to just looking around you. The learner must learn to scan through the options available to them without accidentally triggering any selections, then hold their stare at the thing they want to select. Then they need to ensure that they look away from the selection offered to indicate they have nothing more to say, or make use of pause selections.

Block scanning – by scanning sections (blocks), then when the block is selected, by row/column and finally scanning each item linearly when the row/column is selected.

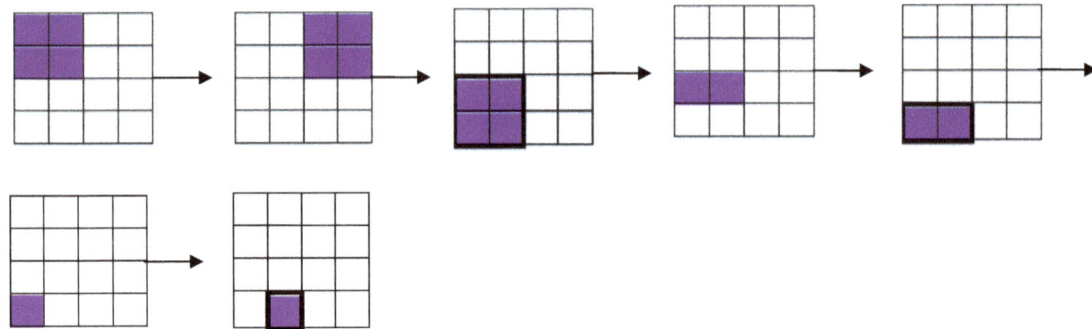

Block scanning pattern

Figure 13.22 An image of 7 squares explaining scanning patterns.

Source: Smartbox, creators of Grid AAC software.

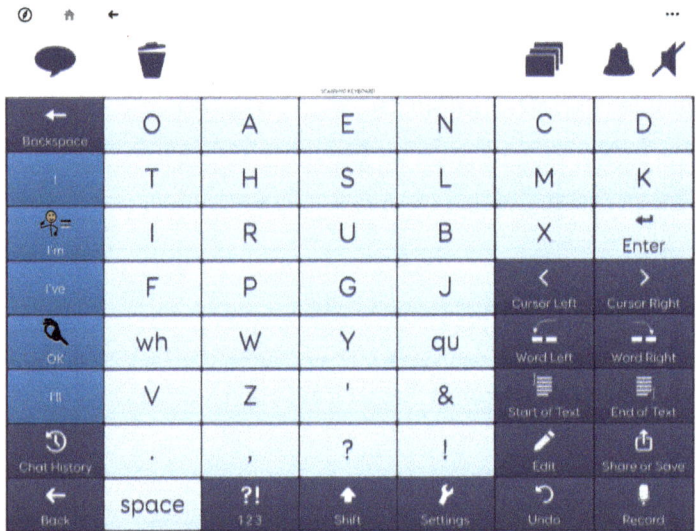

Figure 13.23 An image of a blue on screen keyboard with the letters arranged in frequency order.

Source: Smartbox, creators of Grid AAC software.

When introducing eye pointing as an access method, as with all other access methods, it may be easier to introduce eye pointing to paper-based resources with a communication partner first. The communication partner knows the context of the day, knows when the learner is distracted and will have a better understanding if a mistake has been made, as they have all of the context of the interaction. An electronic AAC aid is not as forgiving as human support when supporting a learner using eye pointing as an access method.

When using eye pointing for communication, many learners use a tool called an E-Tran frame. As you can see in the image below the communication partner holds the frame between themselves and the individual who is eye pointing. Then they say and recall the selections made. In this example the user is literate and is therefore spelling out messages. Your learners are likely to need to use aided language, in the form of symbols.

Figure 13.24 shows different eye pointing, paper-based resources using symbols. These are ones which you can just print and cut out the middle section so you can see the learner's eye point.

The amount of language we can offer the learner when using eye pointing as an access method can be increased by using colour coding. An example of this is the Look2Talk book created by Ace Centre (Figure 13.25).

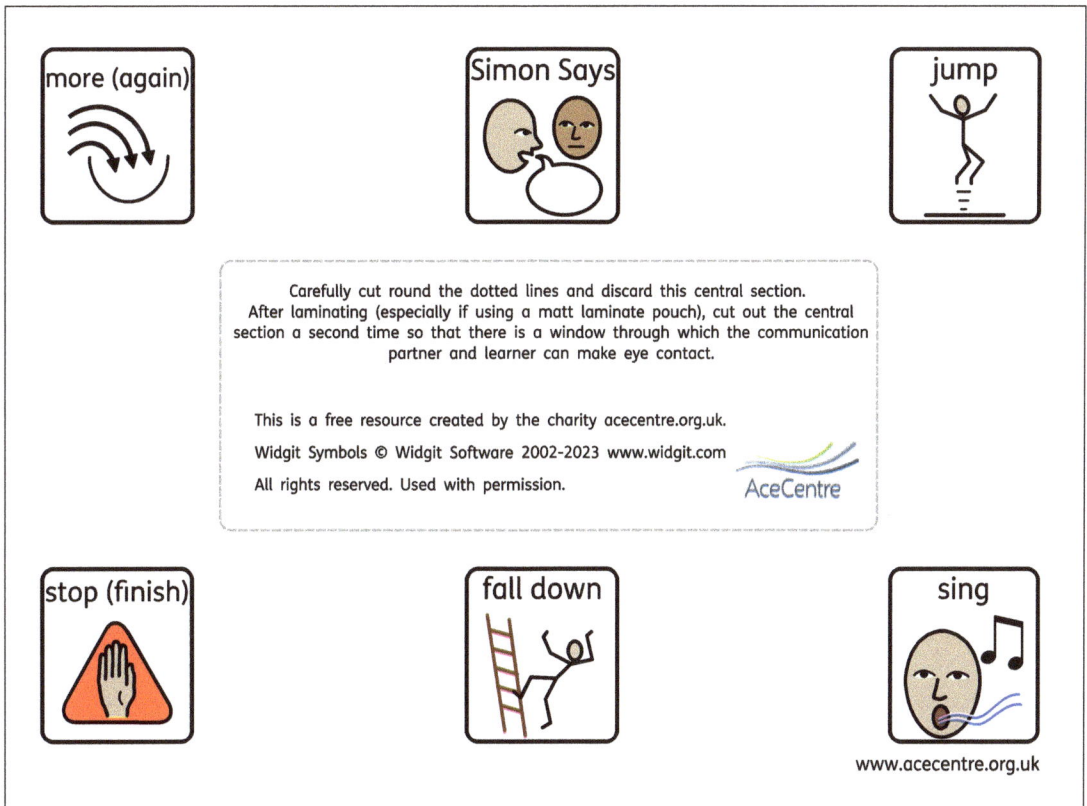

Figure 13.24 Simon Says symbol chart to use through eye pointing.

Source: Created by Ace Centre https://acecentre.org.uk/resources

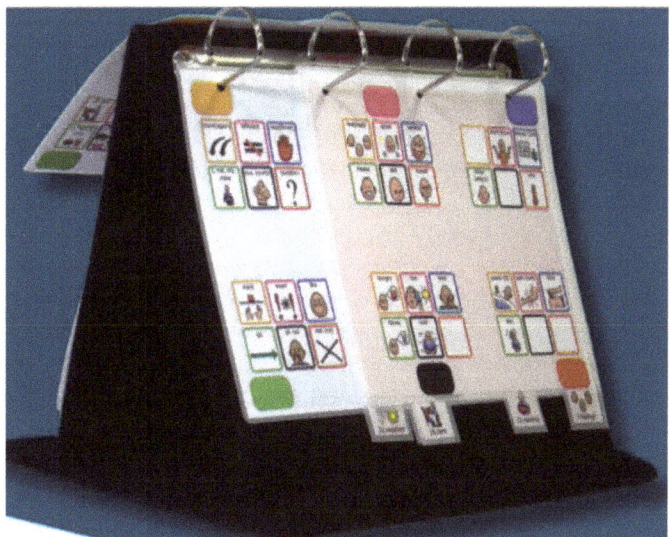

Figure 13.25 Folder back ring binder, stood upright with pages with symbols on.

Source: Created by Ace Centre https://acecentre.org.uk/resources

Eye Gaze with Technology

Eye gaze technology is the use of an eye gaze camera connected to a computer or tablet – for example, Windows tablet or iPad. The eye gaze cameras reflect light from the learner's eyes and use that to read the learner's eye movement across the screen. To select using eye pointing, the learner must dwell their eyes on the target they want to select. Many proficient eye gaze users, apply eye gaze in conjunction with other access methods, such as switch scanning, as using

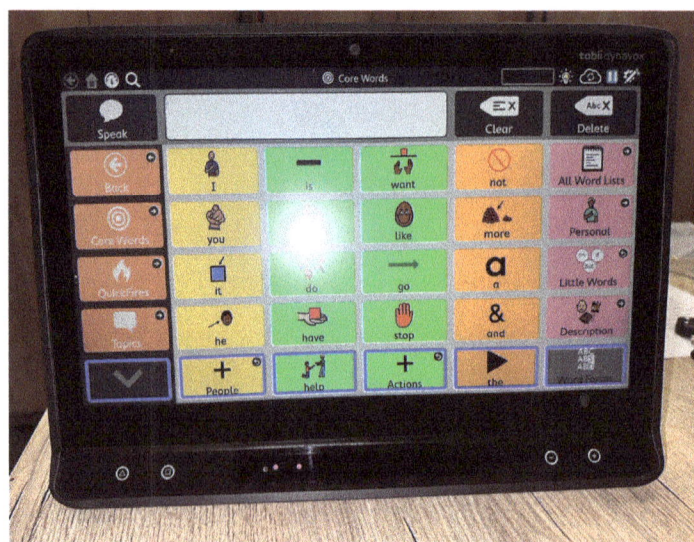

Figure 13.26 Image of an electronic communication aid with symbols on the screen.

Source: Photographed by the author.

your eyes to communicate all day can be visually tiring – the same way that you get visual fatigue when you have been staring at a computer screen all day.

Eye gaze cameras can be separate and connect to the computer, communication aid or tablet via a wired connection, others are inbuilt. When buying an eye gaze camera for a learner it is worthwhile looking into the features of the different cameras. Some are better at compensating for involuntary head movement, reading eye movements when in sunlight and when the learner wears glasses. It's advisable to trial the camera before you buy by asking the company who supplies them to come into school and support you in setting it up for the learner to trial.

Figure 13.26 is an example of an inbuilt camera from Tobii Dynavox.

Cameras come with their own software so you need to check with the company that you are purchasing the eye gaze camera from that the software will work with your device. When looking at eye gaze as an access method for AAC, this is a health need, and any assessment should be led by the learner's speech and language therapist. Many specialist school settings do purchase technology such as eye gaze cameras for learners to use, to develop skills in using this access method, which can then be used for leisure, curriculum access or communication.

When introducing eye gaze technology with learners in your class, it's worthwhile having a go yourself first. That will highlight how challenging controlling a device with eye gaze access can be and will give you a better idea of how to prompt and support your learner.

Sometimes the hesitation to select, by waiting for the eye gaze camera to register where you are looking, may be challenging, as the learner may struggle to hold their stare. If this is the case, the settings can be changed so the learner uses a switch to make the selection once they have looked at the item they want on the screen.

As with all access methods there is an element of skill development in learning to control the computer or tablet with your eyes. There are some skill development tools that could support your learner on their journey, such as Inclusive Technology's Eye Gaze Learning Curve.

Other factors to consider when trying to support a learner with the effective use of eye gaze as an access method are:

Fatigue: The learner may get tired as the day progresses, they may need to close their eyes, they may struggle to maintain their head position or their position in their wheelchair. All these factors linked to fatigue, could impact of the effective use of eye gaze technology. That is why it is important to have an alternative the learner can use, such as access via eye pointing on paper-based resources, or by using scanning (either switch scanning or partner assisted scanning).

Mounting: Eye Gaze cameras need to be a certain height and distance from the learner to be able to read their eyes effectively. The devices that eye gaze cameras are inbuilt into (such as dedicated AAC devices) and devices that an eye gaze camera could connect to (such as a laptop), can be quite heavy and therefore need to be safely mounted. Mounting these devices should be thoroughly risk assessed and advice should be sought around safety regulations for mounting.

Partner support: For a learner to use eye gaze as an access method, it requires dedication and skill from the team around the learner. The team supporting must know how to set up the device, for example, get the camera in the right position. They need to ensure the camera is calibrated to the learner's eyes and trouble shoot any issues.

The Environment: Lighting can affect the use of eye gaze cameras massively. It is worthwhile considering how much natural light is in the classroom and other areas of the school where the learner will be using the eye gaze camera. Will the learner be outside a lot? Will there constantly be other learners leaning over them to look at the screen and confusing the eye gaze camera? These are all factors that you will need to consider if introducing eye gaze as an access method for your learner.

Alternative Mice

For some learners controlling a device with a standard mouse can be difficult. Think now about how you use a mouse when you are accessing a computer. What skills do you need to have to do what you want to do? You will need to understand that when you move the mouse it moves a cursor on the screen of your chosen device. Then you would need enough control to move the mouse to get the cursor over the target you want on the screen. Next is changing your movement to a press on one of the buttons on the mouse to select. How did you know which button to press? Then you may need other movement patterns, depending on what you are trying to do; for example, when highlighting something you would need the combination of a click and drag.

The complex nature of using a standard mouse is why some learners may need alternative mice to enable them to control the given device. Here is a small selection of alternative mice.

When trialling alternative mice, it is important to realise that positioning is key. The position of the device will make the difference between the learner being able to use it effectively or not. Therefore, you may need to consider mounting the device to the learner's wheelchair, using items to stabilise the alternative mouse such as a bean bag or Dycem non-slip matting underneath it.

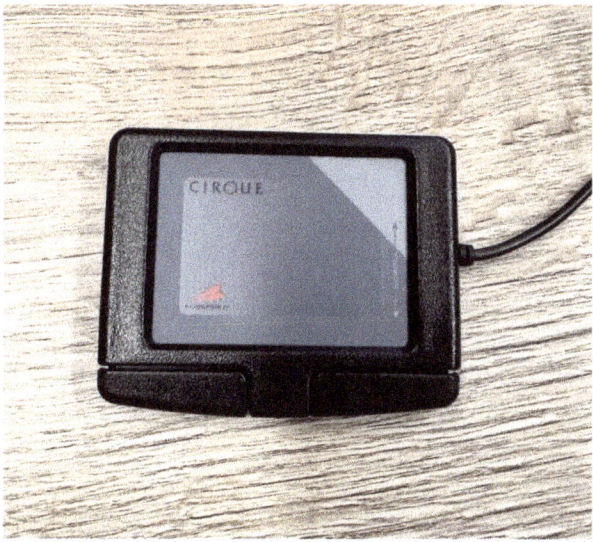

Figure 13.27 A black rectangular touch pad to control a computer.

Source: Photographed by the author.

Touch Pads

Touch pads offer mouse input with minimum movement (Figure 13.27). They generally have buttons on them for left and right clicks and those clicks can often be replicated by the tapping of the sensor as well. People typically see touch pads embedded into laptops. However, having them separate offers greater positioning flexibility to get the best positioning for optimal control for the learner.

Trackballs/Rollerballs (Figures 13.28 and 13.29)

Trackballs require less space, in that the learner doesn't need as much surface space to move the track balls, as the unit itself stays stationary and it is only the ball which moves the cursor across the screen. Track balls are ergonomic to use as they require less movement. You can get them with wired or Bluetooth connection. They can come in a variety of different shapes and sizes. The majority will have buttons on them so learners can press to select a left

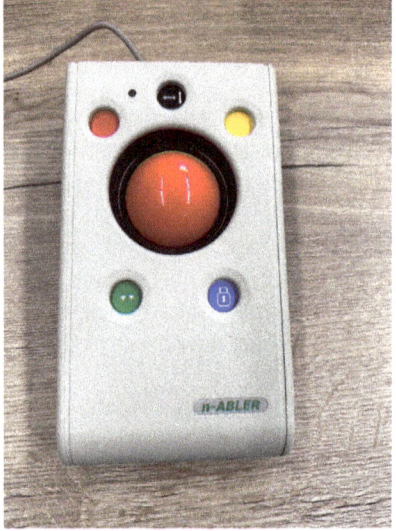

Figure 13.28 A red track ball.
Source: Photographed by the author.

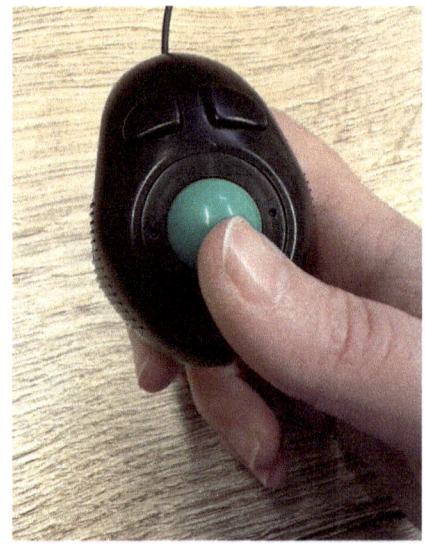

Figure 13.29 A finger mouse being held in a hand. It has a green roller ball on the top.
Source: Photographed by the author.

or right click. Some may need you to plug in additional switches to act as the left and right mouse click.

Joysticks (Figures 13.30 and 13.31)

Again, with joysticks the learner will require less clear space around them as the joystick remains in one place and just the stick controls the movement of the curser on the screen. Joysticks can come in a variety of sizes, and it is worthwhile considering the shape of the joystick tip. Some learners may find it easier to wrap their hand around the stick, others may prefer to rest their hand on top of the tip of the joystick. In that case some learners may benefit from having a ball top to rest their hands on. Some joysticks have selection buttons on them, and others require you to plug in switches and use them to select.

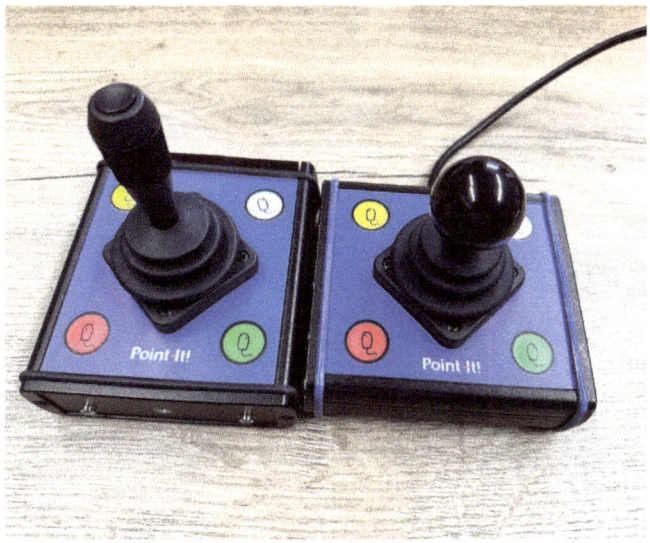

Figure 13.30 Two joysticks.

Source: Photographed by the author.

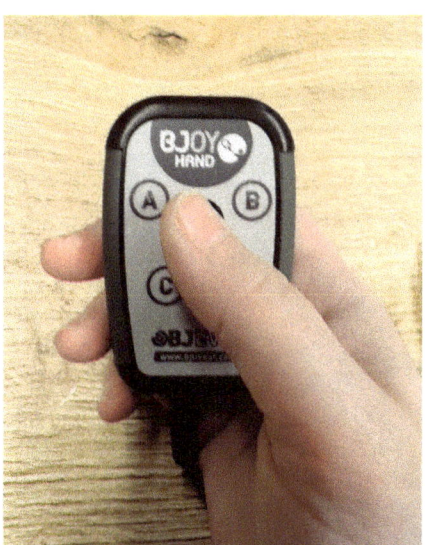

Figure 13.31 A handheld joystick.

Source: Photographed by the author.

Integrated Joysticks

If a learner has a power chair it may be possible that they could use the existing joystick on their chair to control the cursor on a device by using a Bluetooth connection, with a system like the example shown. If you contact the learner's wheelchair service they should be able to advise whether the joystick can have Bluetooth connectors added to allow computer control.

Head Mouse (Figure 13.32)

Head mice can be used for learners who struggle with the physical movement of controlling a mouse with their hands. Head mice are suitable for learners who have good control over their head movement. This access method is not suitable for a learner who struggles to maintain an upright head position. There are different types of head mouse, some of which

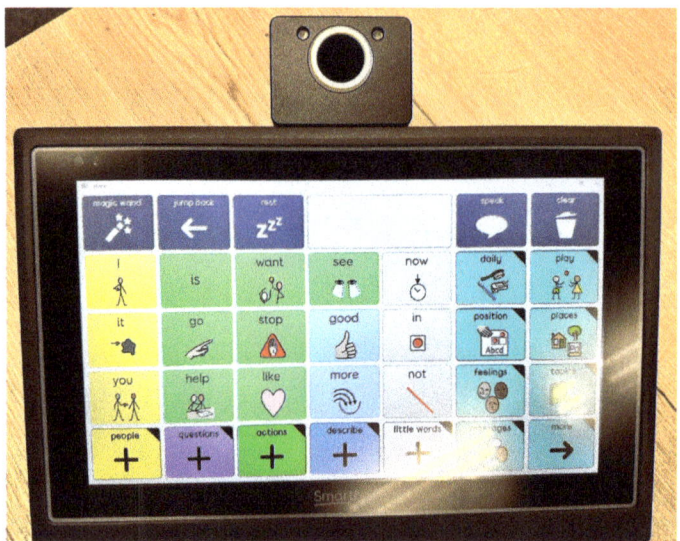

Figure 13.32 An image of an electronic communication aid with a black square box attached to the top.

Source: Photographed by author. SmartBox, creators of Grid AAC software.

work by the learner wearing a reflective sticker on the middle of their glasses, or on their forehead (between the eyes). Then the computer uses that dot to replicate the learner's head movement on the cursor on the screen. Other head mice use technology such as a gyroscope to detect head movement and replicate that movement pattern with the cursor on the screen.

When trialling the effectiveness of alternative mice with your learner, it may also be useful to think about some of the adaptations that can be made within the software, such as changing the mouse, click and pointer settings. Here are some examples of how you could change those settings within Windows software.

Mouse Settings (Figures 13.33, 13.34 and 13.35)

Here you can change settings, such as the mouse pointer speed and style. Sometimes slowing this down helps learners to track where the cursor is as it moves across the screen. Likewise, some learners may benefit from a larger cursor to help them locate it on the screen. Other

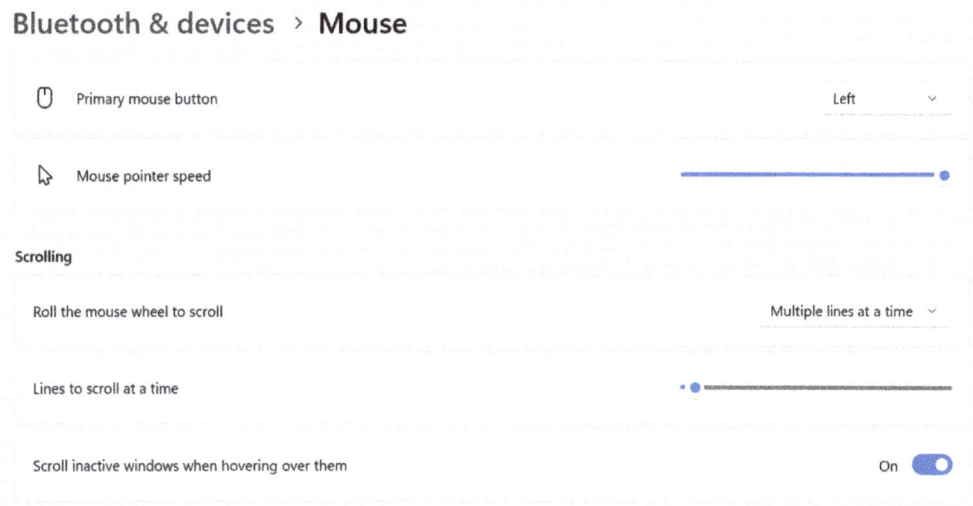

Figure 13.33 A screen shot of Windows Bluetooth and Devices > Mouse settings.

Source: Screen captures from Windows 10 PC accessibility settings.

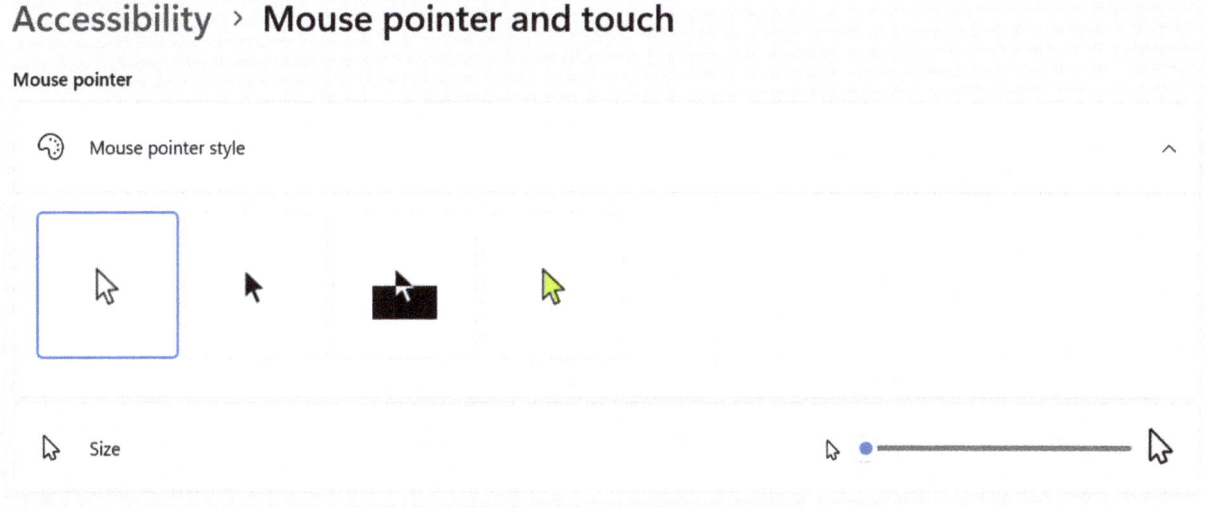

Figure 13.34 A screen shot of Windows Mouse pointer and touch settings.

Source: Windows 10 PC accessibility settings.

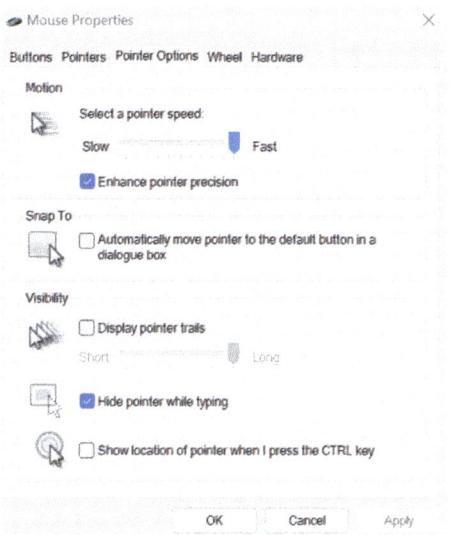

Figure 13.35 A screen shot of Windows Mouse Properties.

Source: Windows 10 PC accessibility settings.

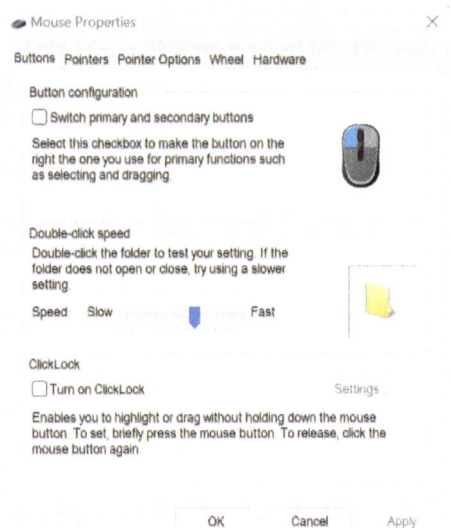

Figure 13.36 A screenshot of the Windows Mouse Properties dialog box.

Source: Screen shot capture from Windows 10 PC accessibility settings.

features such as creating a trail behind the cursor can also be added via the settings displayed. This makes it visually easier to access and supports learners in understanding which direction they are moving the mouse.

Click Settings

Within these settings you can change click settings, such as no longer requiring a double click or changing the speed required for a double click. This is helpful for learners who may struggle with control to double click a mouse.

You can also set features such as ClickLock to make highlighting easier, as it removes the need for the click and drag, which many learners with physical disabilities find challenging.

Conclusion

This chapter has looked at how learners with physical disabilities can access devices and access paper-based resources with the support from a communication partner. Although the focus of this book is aided language and AAC in the classroom, it is worthwhile noting that finding an effective access method for a learner with physical disabilities can open up their world and give them the independence they desire, not just for communication via AAC, but also for access to education and leisure. Technology constantly evolves, and the response of 'they can't do that because they can't touch it/hold it', is no longer acceptable. Where there is a will there is a way. Never be scared to ask the question, how can we support the learner to achieve this? Technology is not a magic wand, and there will always be a journey around skill development when considering different access methods but if the access method allows the learner to achieve their goal, then the hard work and effort will have been worth it!

The following chapter considers the importance of goal setting to steer your learners' journey towards autonomous communication using aided language/AAC.

Bibliography

Burkhart, L. (2018). Stepping Stones to Switch Access. *Perspectives of the ASHA Special Interest Groups*, 3(12), pp.33–44. doi: https://doi.org/10.1044/persp3.sig12.33

Integrating Academic, Communication and Motor Programs for Students with Significant Disabilities. (n.d.). Available at: www.communicationmatrix.org/Uploads/Posts/8259/RedYellowGreenDirections.pdf [Accessed 14 Jan. 2024].

Cotter, C., Porter, G., & Burkhart, L. (2016, July). Course manual for teaching movements for communication. Westminster, MD: Author.

Goodwyn, S. W., Acredolo, L. P., & Brown, C. A. (2000). Impact of symbolic gesturing on early language development. Journal of Nonverbal Behavior, 24(2), pp.81–103.

Switch Progression Learning Journeys Road Map. (n.d.). Available at: https://atinternetmodules.org/storage/ocali-ims-sites/ocali-ims-atim/documents/Inclusive_TLC_switch-progression-road-map.pdf

Pace. (n.d.). *Sevenstages*. [online] Available at: https://thepacecentre.org/sevenstages/ [Accessed 14 Jan. 2024].

www.helpkidzlearn.com. (n.d.). HKL Games & Activities – Shop | HelpKidzLearn. [online] Available at: www.helpkidzlearn.com/shop/online-software/games-and-activities

www.project-core.com. (n.d.). *Project Core – A Stepping-Up Technology Implementation Grant Directed by the Center for Literacy and Disability Studies*. [online] Available at: www.project-core.com/

14 Assessment and Target Setting

This book so far has considered good practice in implementing aided language in the classroom. It is worth considering that learners in the classroom have a unique set of skills and understanding, so practices put in place should be bespoke to their individual needs and language development. Goal setting is an important aspect when considering where the learner is currently working and taking steps to move them forward and make progress. It is important to ensure this is carried out in a multidisciplinary manner to be most successful, with the whole team working with the learner towards the same goals. This should include parents and carers, teachers and support staff, speech and language therapists, and any other relevant professionals – for example respite workers who work with the learner outside of the school and home contexts. Goals should be written down and agreed by the team around the learner.

The biggest barrier to successfully writing goals for learners who have AAC systems is that staff, both teachers and therapists, don't feel unsure in the implementation of AAC and lack confidence in this field. Resources signposted in this chapter give examples you can use in your own practice to better support the learners within your classroom.

When considering goal setting, assessments play heavily in identifying where a learner is currently working. Goal setting fits into the assessment plan, do review cycle, through identifying a learner's needs, planning how to meet these, put plan in place, monitoring and adjusting as necessary, and reviewing how the support is meeting the learner's needs. This enables you to review goals over shorter as well as longer lengths of time. The goal being that the learner will be able to say whatever they want to say, to whoever they want to say it, whenever they want to say it (Porter, 2018). Recording observations is a key component when working with learners who use aided language/AAC, because their communication is not physically recorded by the learner on paper as you would see in written tasks. Due to this, it is vital those working with the learners can compile accurate observations. Burkhart and Porter (2010) offer a range of examples of how observations could be recorded in a variety of ways.

There are three key elements required for successful goal writing, including do, condition, and criterion statements. All these elements are included in well-written goals.

1. *Do statements* include what the learner is expected to do, identifying the specific skill the learner is working on.
2. *Condition statements* provide information regarding the setting and context where the learner will be practising the skill.
3. *Criterion statements* indicate how the learner's success will be measured.

An acronym which you will often see used when setting goals and targets is being SMART, which means goals are:

- *Specific* to the individual learner, and not broad.
- *Measurable* so that progress can be tracked.
- *Attainable* using verbs such as the learner 'will …' These should be achievable for the learner.
- *Relevant* considering the learner's skills.
- *Timely* with a clear ending by when they should be achieved.

Regarding setting communication targets, these can be specific in several different ways, including:

- *By context*, for example whether the task is structured, specific to an activity, time of day, setting, or occurring in more natural conversation.
- *By level of prompting*, for example whether the prompts are direct, indirect or independent.

- *Quantifiable*, a percentage – for example, 80 per cent of the time.
- *By frequency*, for example 5 times a day, 3 times during a given activity. To ensure this is monitored, data collection plays a key role.
- *Linguistically*, for example whether at a single word level or sentence level.

The Education, Health and Care Plans (EHCP) process and corresponding annual reviews are great ways to set and review goals and targets, however these are not in place for all learners with Speech Language and Communication Needs (SLCN), who benefit from aided language/AAC in the classroom, so it is important to have processes where these learners also can have goals set and reviewed.

When considering appropriate goals for learners it is important to ensure these are meaningful for the learner.

> A goal which requires a child to comment, ask a question or request at a specific time may in fact lead to practices which reinforce the child's concept that communication is a meaningless task, rather than a powerful personal tool I can use to communicate my own messages.
> (Burkhart and Porter, 2010)

Burkhart and Porter (2010) stress the importance of flexibility to allow the learner to have opportunities to say what they want to say when they want to say it, and this approach should focus on a range of communicative functions (for example requesting, commenting, instructing, negating) incorporated into everyday, real life situations. This contrasts with basing goals around what someone else may want the learner to say, in artificial contexts, based on the communication partner's agenda and within a testing situation. Goals can be measured without having to formally test a learner.

The National Curriculum (DfE, 2014), pre-key stage national standards (DfE, 2018) and engagement scales (DfE, 2020) are all documents created by the DfE, and cover content to be taught at different ability levels. However, unlike stereotypical learning, for example counting to 10, these do not reference progression for learners with Speech Language and Communication Needs who use aided language/AAC. Due to this lack of guidance, setting relevant goals for learners who use aided language/AAC can feel overwhelming. Fear not, there are several examples of documentation which can be used to set goals for this specific group of learners. There is a vast array of examples, and within this chapter we focus on the Dynamic AAC Goals Grid-3 (Tobii Dynavox, 2023) and the Communication Matrix (Rowland, 2013).

Dynamic AAC Goals Grid-3

This is an assessment tool used to assess, plan, implement and track goals for learners who have AAC systems in place across a spectrum of abilities. Dynamic AAC Goals Grid-3 allows the individual to assess and then re-assess the learner's current communication skills. This can inform the development of a plan and goals to develop a learner's independence when communicating. It enables the individual to see the bigger picture when setting goals, considering current as well as future goals.

This document considers a range of elements required to ultimately achieve fully autonomous, independent communication. It includes checklists corresponding to Janice Light's communicative competencies (1989), including linguistic, operational social and strategic competence. It identifies these as:

- *Linguistic competency* as expressing and understanding language, learning, and using vocabulary. This also encompasses literacy elements, including reading, writing, and spelling.
- *Operational competency* as the ability to maintain, navigate, and operate the AAC system using the learner's chosen access method.
- *Social competency* as the ability to communicate effectively and in socially appropriate ways.
- *Strategic competency* as the ability to use strategies to overcome or minimise the functional limitations of AAC. It gives the communication partners a vehicle to assess the learner's communication strengths and weaknesses to support the identification of appropriate goals.

This chain of cues used within DAGG allows the individual to identify the next steps for the learner to work towards independence.

This chain of cues includes:

- Natural cues: Expect communication, lean forward and use facial expressions to show interest
- Indirect cues: Motion towards the communication device with your hand
- Direct cues: Ask opinion questions, for example 'What do you think?' and 'What do you know about ... ?'

Starting with the least amount of cueing, if the learner does not respond after a pause, the communication partner can then progress to a more direct cue.

The Dynamic AAC Goals Grid-3 identifies the steps to independence as an ability continuum, including Emergent, Emergent Transitional, Context Dependent, Transitional Independent and Independent. It is worth noting the learner may be working at a different level for different competencies.

Due to this, the smallest of progress towards independence can be identified and documented to set relevant, achievable goals. These will be short-term goals, but longer-term goals are 'based on projections of future opportunities, needs, constraints, and capabilities resulting from instruction within those competencies' (Buekelman and Miranda, 2005).

The Dynamic AAC Goals Grid-3 is broken down into the following steps:

1. Identify the communication ability level of the learner.
2. Review goals in each competency area and mark the goals that have already been met to identify potential competency areas to focus on.
3. Determine the level of support needed for each target goal required.
4. Identify implementation and teaching techniques.
5. Fill out the implementation planning and goals progress report included.
6. Fill out the progress summary on the first page to give an overview.

> **Discussion Point!**
>
> - Have a look at the Dynamic AAC Goals Grid-3, which can be accessed here: www.tobiidynavox.com/pages/dagg-3-resources (you will need to enter your email to do so).
> - Choose a learner you are supporting who uses aided language/AAC. Can you identify where they are currently working and use this to inform the setting of appropriate goals?

Communication Matrix

The Communication Matrix is another tool that can be used to record and document a learner's communication skills. Information can be gathered from observations and interactions with the learner using an AAC system. The tool was created to help professionals understand the communication, progress and needs of the learner.

The Matrix assesses the level of communication shown by learners, including those who use AAC Systems. It can be used to assess the earliest of communicators, typically working on the Engagement Scale Model (2020). It records a range of communicative behaviours, both unintentional and intentional as well as pre-symbolic and symbolic language. This can be used for all ages.

The Matrix includes Seven Levels of Communication, described below:

Level 1: Pre-Intentional Behaviour

This level covers behaviours which the learner does not have control over and is not using these to communicate intentionally. Learners have not yet learnt that their behaviours have an impact on the behaviour of others. It is the role of the communication partner at this stage to interpret a learner's behaviour to identify their needs. Examples of behaviour at this stage includes body language, e.g. turning their head away from a stimulus; facial expressions, e.g. smiling; vocalisations, e.g. crying; or eye gaze, e.g. tracking something across the room. They exhibit these behaviours without knowing that the communication partner will respond to these. The learner may cry to show they are hungry, thirsty, or upset. They may also smile or make happy sounds when they are happy and content.

Level 2: Intentional Behaviour

This level covers behaviours which the learner does have control over and is beginning to use these intentionally. They are learning that their behaviours have an impact on the communication partner. The learner will communicate using their body language, facial expressions, vocalisations and eye gaze. The learner is realising these behaviours will gain attention. They will begin to communicate their needs, for example, they are learning if they cry this may be interpreted as them being upset, hungry or thirsty. If they smile and laugh this will show the communication partner they are happy. They are also learning they can protest if they do not want to do something.

Level 3: Unconventional Communication

This level covers communication, which is pre-symbolic, that the learner uses. Their communication does not yet include the use of symbols. The learner will continue to communicate using body language, facial expressions, vocalisations and eye gaze, as well as the use of gestures, for example, leading the communication partner to something they want or pointing to people or objects. They have learnt that they will often get what they want by exhibiting these behaviours. Learners may exhibit challenging behaviour at times as a means of communicating to get their needs met as they do not yet have a formal way of communicating these.

Level 4: Conventional Communication

This level covers learners who are using conventional, pre-symbolic means to intentionally communicate. Behaviours are classed as pre-symbolic due to not including the use of symbols, however, are now conventional in nature as the behaviours exhibited are socially acceptable. Communicative behaviours at this level include pointing, nodding, or shaking their head, waving, hugging, and intentionally looking at the communication partner and object they want. The learner will also continue to use vocalisations to communicate. The learner has learnt that specific gestures are understood by the communication partner to mean something specific. An example of this may be pointing to a toy they wish to play with, they know that the communication partner will interpret this as them being interested in the object. The learner may use different vocalisations and gestures with different communication partners. For example, an unfamiliar communication partner compared to caregivers. The learner may continue to exhibit some challenging behaviour; however, they have now learnt alternative ways of communicating which the communication partner will understand. They may now have gained more appropriate behaviours to protest, for example dropping to the floor to communicate they do not want to do something.

Level 5: Concrete Symbols

This level covers Symbolic language which can be used to represent an object to communicate. These concrete symbols look like what they represent. This can include pictures, objects of reference (e.g., a cup to represent a drink), iconic gestures (e.g., waving at a communication partner to say hello or goodbye), and sounds (for example, saying 'mmmmmm' to represent mum). There is a shared understanding between the learner and communication partner about what these symbols represent.

Level 6: Abstract Symbols

This level covers more abstract symbols, including speech, sign language, braille, and written words. At this level the symbols are described as abstract as they are not physically like what they represent. The learner may also begin to use an AAC System to communicate. They will point to 1 symbol or create a single sign to get their message across, however they may begin to combine 2 symbols together, for example pointing to 'car' and 'go'. The learner will use core words, for example, asking for 'more' of a given activity.

Level 7. Language Levels

At this level learners use symbols, both concrete and abstract in combination, for example, in order to create 2 and 3 word sentence strings (e.g., 'want mum', 'want more crisps' 'help me open', 'stop car' and 'I like bubbles'). The learner understands these sentences and basic grammatical concepts, for example, the right order to combine objects (e.g., 'like grapes' rather than 'grapes like'). At this level the learner will use core words, including verbs and adjectives in combination with nouns (e.g., 'play train' and 'big ball'). This can be built into longer sentence strings (e.g., 'want play train' or 'like big ball'). The learner will continue to make use of non-verbal communication to support their message (e.g., the learner may point to the trainset or ball when communicating about them, to show they would like these objects). This gives the communication partner further information about what it is the learner is communicating.

You will often experience some overlap between levels when assessing pupils as these can occur simultaneously. The learner may communicate in different ways dependent on the environment, who they are communicating with, or what they are communicating.

The Matrix identifies the 4 key reasons to communicate as: to refuse things they don't want; to obtain things they want; to engage in social interaction; and to provide or seek information. The Matrix (Rowland, 2013, pp. 2–3) identifies these as follows:

REFUSE

- Expresses discomfort.
- Protests
- Refuses or rejects something.

OBTAIN

- Expresses comfort.
- Continues an action.
- Obtains more of something.
- Requests more of an action.
- Requests a new action.
- Requests more of an object.
- Makes choices.
- Requests a new object.
- Requests objects that are absent.

SOCIAL

- Expresses interest in other people.
- Attracts attention.
- Requests attention.
- Shows affection.
- Greets people.
- Offers things or shares.
- Directs someone's attention to something.
- Uses polite social forms.

> *INFORMATION*
>
> - Answers 'yes' and 'no' questions.
> - Ask questions.
> - Names things or people.
> - Makes comments.
>
> The Communication Matrix is free for anyone to use; it can be found here: www.communicationmatrix.org/Matrix/About#

By using the Matrix online, you can manage information to identify specifically how the learner is currently communicating and identify specific goals for the learner to work towards. The Matrix enables the communication partner to track progress over time. This can be shared with parents and carers, supporting the creation of a holistic picture about how the learner is communicating in different environments and contexts.

An example of a completed Matrix for a learner can be seen in this image.

Figure 14.1 clearly shows at a glance the level at which the learner is currently communicating and their next steps. For example, in the Matrix the learner has surpassed level 1 and 2 and is now working within level 3. The learner has mastered refusing and rejecting. Their next step would be requesting more of an action. The Matrix identified this step as including the elements below:

Body language

- Whole body movement.
- Arm/hand movement.
- Leg movement.

Early sounds

- Cooing, squealing, laughing.

Facial expressions

- Smiling

Visual

- Looking at the communication partner.

Simple gesture

- Taking the communication partner's hand.
- Touching the communication partner.
- Reaching towards or taps the communication partner.

The learner is not required to use all of these strategies to request more; for example, a learner may have no control over their movement or be unable to produce sound. Looking at the elements above, one specific goal may be for the learner to work on using a simple gesture – for example, taking the communication partner's hand to guide them. To make the goal SMART this can be written as follows: "Xxx will be able to take the communication partner's hand to an object to request more of an activity for 5 activities throughout the school day independently." This is easily quantifiable and can thus be tracked to record progress. By recording what activities the learner is requesting, patterns can be identified, e.g., the learner may solely be asking for more bubbles by leading a communication partner's hand, but using strategies from previous levels for different activities. Observations will also be valuable to identify how independent the learner is and track this progress as the learner may be receiving direct or indirect cues to achieve the goal. This can then be marked on the Matrix whether it is an emerging skill or mastered.

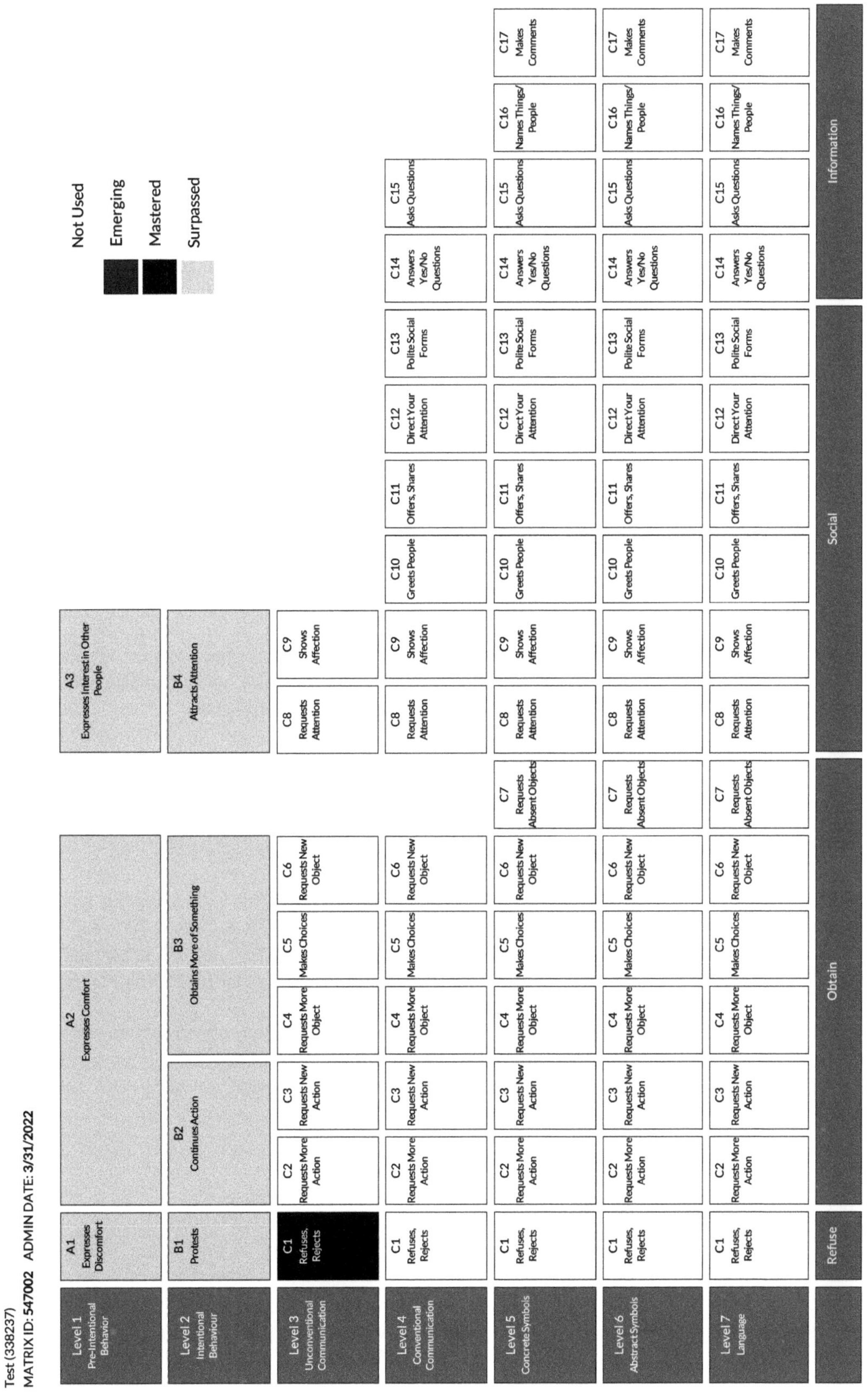

Figure 14.1 This image shows a table in grey and white.

Source: Created using the online version of the Communication Matrix.

Looking at the Matrix, another learner may be working at level 6 to request more of an object. At this level elements include the use of abstract symbols:

- Spoken word.
- Sign language.
- Writing
- Braille
- Abstract 3D symbols.
- Abstract 2D symbols.

A relevant goal at this level may be: "Xxx will combine the symbol 'more' and a relevant verb to request more of an action when playing during an activity of their choosing 80% of the time with indirect cues".

As with the goal above, this is achievable and quantifiable; however, this is not simply counting how many times throughout the day. Instead, this will require observation by the communication partner to identify how often the learner is combining 'more' and the action and the level of prompting required. This goal has stated that the communication partner is able to offer indirect cues, rather than expecting the learner to carry out the task independently. This breaks the goal down into smaller steps so that it is more easily achievable for the learner.

> **Discussion Point!**
>
> - Take a look at the overview of the Matrix included in this chapter.
> - Can you identify where one of your learners may be working?
> - What may be relevant goals for them to achieve a given step?

Explore the online version of the Communication Matrix available at www.communicationmatrix.org/ You can download a PDF version of the tool for free, and profile up to five learners using the online tool. You will then need to pay for additional saved assessments.

Conclusion

This chapter has explored two useful tools which can be used to set goals for a learner who uses aided language/AAC and track progress using these tools. They give a clear indication of the language development of the learner and can be used as a resource to illustrate progress within a learner's language-development journey. These are both free resources to download, and can support your learner towards autonomous communication.

In the following chapter we consider the importance of gaining pupil voice within the school setting. For learners with SLCN, who use aided language/AAC, it is of extra importance that these learners have the opportunity to express their autonomous thoughts within the safety of the school environment.

Bibliography

Beukelman, D. and Mirenda, P. (2005). *Augmentative and alternative communication: Supporting children and adults with complex communication needs*, 3rd ed., Baltimore, MD: Paul H. Brookes.

Burkhart, L. and Porter, G. (2010). *Writing IEP goals and objectives for authentic communication – for children who have complex communication needs*. Available at: Writing IEP Goals 10 and 16 rev (lindaburkhart.com) (Accessed: 14 January 2024).

Department for Education and Department of Health (2014). *National Curriculum*. Available at: www.gov.uk/government/collections/national-curriculum (Accessed: 14 January 2024).

Department for Education and Department of Health (2018). *Pre-key stage 1: pupils working below the national curriculum assessment standard*. Available at: www.gov.uk/government/publications/pre-key-stage-1-standards/pre-key-stage-1-pupils-working-below-the-national-curriculum-assessment-standard (Accessed: 14 January 2024).

Department for Education and Department of Health (2020). *The engagement model*. Available at: The engagement model (publishing.service.gov.uk) (Accessed: 14 January 2024).

Light, J. (1989). Toward a Definition of Communicative Competence for Individuals Using Augmentative and Alternative Communication Systems. *Augmentative and Alternative Communication*, 5(2), pp.137–144.

Porter, G. (2018). *Pragmatic organisation dynamic display communication books: Introductory workshop*. Melb: Cerebral Palsy Education Centre.

Rowland, C. (2013). *Communication matrix for parents and professionals*. Available at: Communication Matrix Handbook 01-07-2013 (Accessed: 14 January 2024).

Tobii Dynavox (2023). *Dynamic AAC Goals Grid-3*. Available at: https://us.tobiidynavox.com/products/dagg-3 (Accessed: 14 January 2024).

15 Opportunities: Pupil Voice

Pupil voice, in the context of education, refers to the active and meaningful participation of learners in the decision-making processes and educational experiences that directly affect them. It is the recognition that learners have valuable insights, opinions, and perspectives that can contribute to improving the quality of their learning environment.

Pupil voice involves creating opportunities for students to express their thoughts, ideas, concerns, and preferences, whether they are related to curriculum, school policies, or extra-curricular activities. Fostering pupil voice empowers learners, promotes a sense of ownership in their education, and fosters a more inclusive and learner-centered approach to schooling. But what does pupil voice look like in practice for learners with significant Speech, Language and Communication Needs (SCLN)?

In the chapter 'More Than Just the Freedom of Speech' we have already looked in detail at the legislation in place to support children to be able to express themselves.

> Children have a right to receive and impart information, to express an opinion and to have that opinion taken into account in any matters affecting them from the early years. Their views should be given due weight according to their age, maturity and capability.
> The United Nations Convention on the Rights of the Child 1989 (Articles 12 and 13)

The government continued to drive this message with the SEND Code of Practice and the SEND review.

> In 2001, the SEN Code of Practice proposed the concept of 'pupil participation' this consolidated the idea of Pupil Voice in education. 'The right of children with special educational needs to be involved in making decisions and exercising choices.' The legislation highlights the importance of the learner's 'voice' being heard and the need for the learner to participate in decisions about their own lives, ready to take their place in society. The SEN Code of Practice set clear guidelines that the local authority must provide the opportunity for the learner to share 'views, wishes and feelings ... participating as fully as possible in decisions' and being provided with the information and support necessary to enable participation in those discussions.
>
> The Revised SEN Code of practice (2015) echoed the 2001 SEN Code of practice, reiterating pupil participation in decision making by involving them in discussions and actively supporting them to 'contributing to needs assessments, developing and reviewing Education, Health and Care Plans (EHCP)'.

> The SEND review 2022: Right Support, Right Place, Right Time, continues to confirm that the young person's voice should be central in decisions about their education and life. It outlined the introduction of consistent standards for 'co-production and communication with children, young people and their families so that they are engaged in the decision-making process around the support that they receive and the progress they are making.'

The danger zone is that pupil voice becomes tokenistic, as educators are aware of the need to seek the opinion of the learner but struggle with how to achieve that when the learner has SLCN.

DOI: 10.4324/9781003410836-15

> **Discussion Point!**
> - What does pupil voice currently look like in your school for a learner with Speech, Language and Communication Needs?
> - When is pupil voice sought? Is it all day every day, or is it just for key events such as annual review meetings of the learner's educational health care plans (EHCP)?

In most cases pupil voice is sought around the time of reviewing educational support. It is essential that educators and stakeholders actively listen to and respect the voices of learners, ensuring that the annual review process is a collaborative effort aimed at enhancing the learner's educational experience and well-being. The idea is that the learner has some say around what provision they will receive by sharing their thoughts and opinions around their current provision. Learners may join the annual review meeting; prepare a presentation about things they like or don't like, or maybe record a short video to be shared with stakeholders in the meeting. At other times the learner's teacher or another member of classroom staff will advocate for them in the meeting. However, advocates often find themselves limited in their ability to fully represent the thoughts and intentions of the learner and, despite their best efforts, are only able to offer an approximation of the learner's thoughts and feelings.

In 2021 Sharma Pooja published a paper which looked at barriers to pupil voice in the EHCP review process (Figure 15.1). In this study, 36 SEND professionals from local authorities and 16 SEND professionals from specialist schools within England were asked their views on eliciting pupil voice through an online-based questionnaire, with a particular focus on the barriers they experience. This was then followed up with six in-depth semi structured interviews.

The findings identify two distinct categories of barriers:

- The barriers relating to children and young people that inhibit their ability to express their views meaningfully.
- The barriers relating to professionals that impede on their ability to elicit views meaningfully within their role.

The image highlights the barriers for children and young people and for professionals identified during the semi-structured interviews.

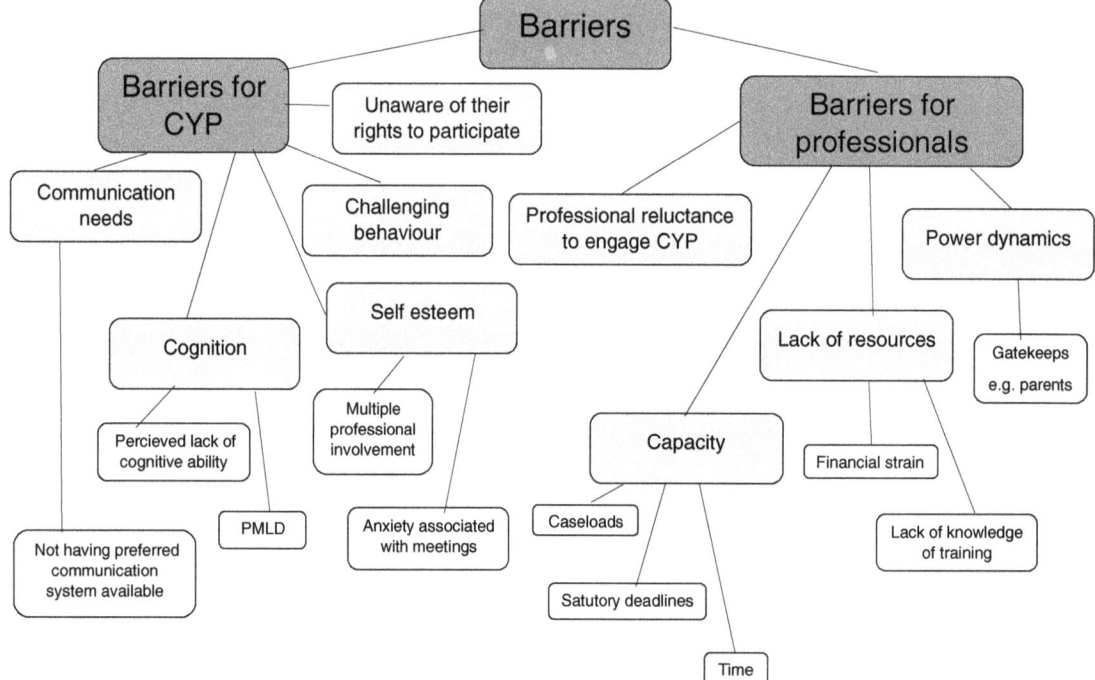

Figure 15.1 This image shows a flowchart of barriers to AAC.

Source: Created by author, adapted from Pooja (2021).

Notes: CYP = child or young person. PMLD = profound and multiple learning difficulties. AAC = augmentative and alternative communication.

This research highlighted some interesting points around barriers for the educator and the child or young person. If we look at the barriers below, it is clear that more information about the learner is required.

Communication Needs: Does the learner have access to aided language to express themselves and have they been taught what that aided language means via aided language input/modelling, so they understand the language available to them?

Cognition: Children classed as having profound and multiple learning difficulties (PMLD) were listed in this category. Learners classed as being PMLD often have complex physical disabilities, too; therefore, is it more that their access method has not yet been found? Alternative access methods are discussed in an earlier chapter.

Challenging Behaviour: Is the learner displaying challenging behaviour due to not having means to communicate their feelings with verbal or aided language?

Self-esteem: If the learner does not have the means to communicate then we know from the research discussed in the chapter that '[m]ore than the Freedom of Speech', there is a higher risk of the learner developing mental health problems.

Unaware of their right to participate: Educational settings inherently have a power imbalance where learners are often given instructions and feedback, with very limited opportunities for them to participate in sharing their thoughts and opinions. This is something that we could be doing all day, every day, so learners know that their opinions are welcomed. Then when we are asking for their opinions in more formal settings, such as in annual review meetings, the concept does not seem alien to the learner.

Aided Language Displays

Gaining learner's opinions can be as simple as having aided language displays/communication charts around the educational setting, so learners have aided language at hand to share their opinions.

The display being there all the time and the language options available invite the learner to participate in sharing their opinion. Without having aided language available, gaining pupil voice would likely be done with closed questioning, only allowing the learner to respond with a yes or no. The goal is autonomous communication, not just answering questions. It is by promoting the autonomy that we achieve true pupil voice and set the learner up to be successful, autonomous communicators.

There are numerous freely available commenting charts that you can download, print and use (Figure 15.2). By having these aided language displays around the environment, there is an inherent expectation for the learner to communicate with you, and for the staff to also be using the aided language displays to model the aided language to the learners in context, rather than a forced interaction.

Once learners become proficient with expressing themselves using aided language displays, it can then be assumed that you will gain a true representation of pupil voice when you ask their opinions around things which affect their life.

Another example of an aided language display is the EHCP commenting chart Figure 15.3. This can be used to gain pupil voice for the learner's annual review of their Education Health Care plan.

Another effective way of gaining a learner's opinion on something is to use a rating scale (Figure 15.4). Once meaning has been attributed to the different colours/faces, a learner can point with their fingers, fists or eyes to the section of the scale that they wish to select to express their opinion on something.

Opportunities: Pupil Voice

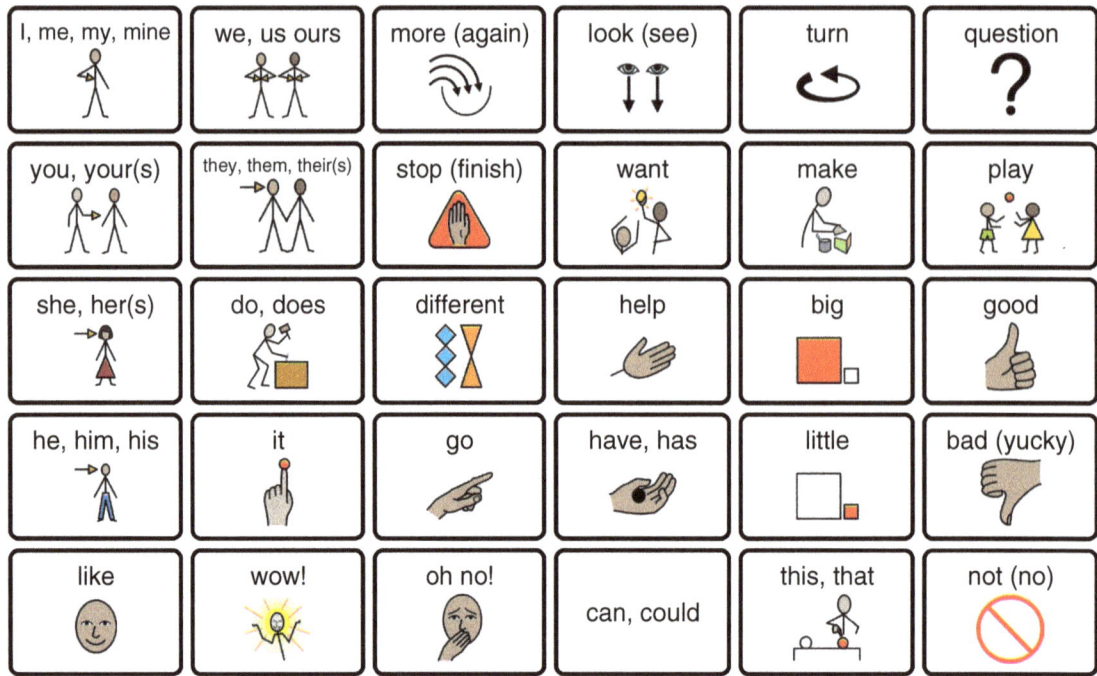

Figure 15.2 Image of 30 symbols with the title core words.

Source: Created by Ace Centre. https://acecentre.org.uk/resources/core

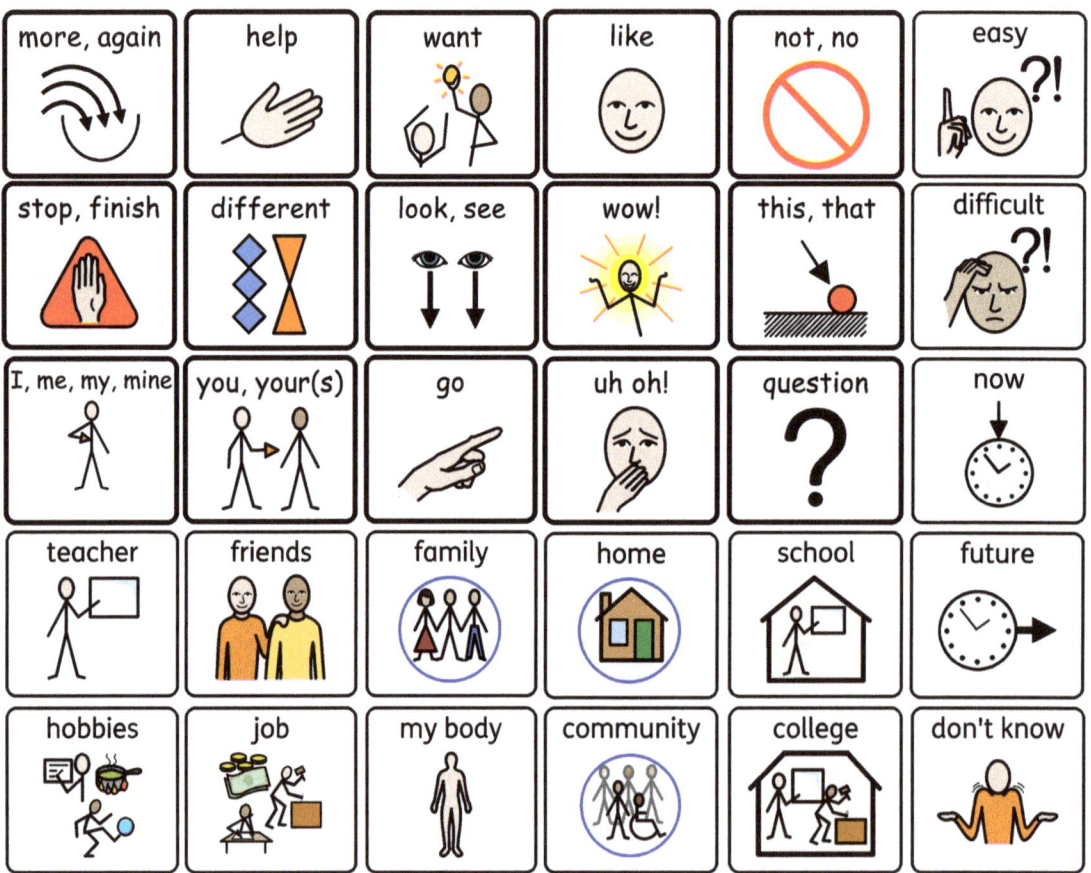

Figure 15.3 Image of 30 symbol EHCP commenting chart.

Source: Created by Ace Centre. https://acecentre.org.uk/resources/core

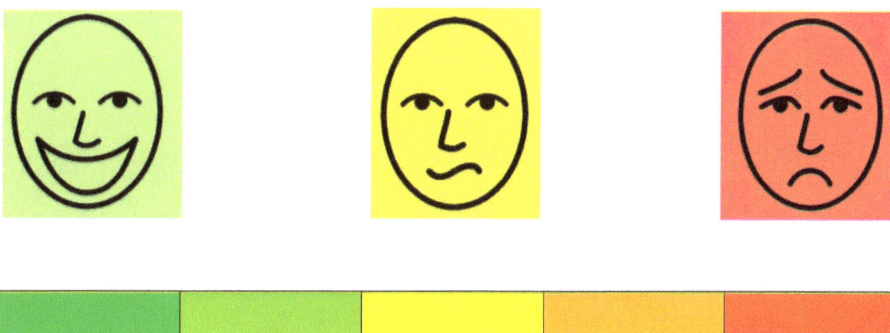

Figure 15.4 This image shows green, yellow, red faces.

Source: Created by Ace Centre https://acecentre.org.uk/resources/core Widgit Symbols © Widgit Software Ltd 2002–2023. www.widgit.com

Talking Mats

Another effective tool is called Talking Mats (Figure 15.5). Talking Mats is a communication tool designed to support learners with various communication difficulties, including those with cognitive impairments, language disorders, or limited verbal abilities. It consists of a set of picture cards and a mat with symbols around specific topics or categories. A communication partner will present the learner with different symbols and ask the learner how they feel about what that symbol represents with open questioning, for example, 'you like it', 'you are not sure' and 'you don't like it'. Then the learner will place the card on the mat in relation to the heading symbols: like, not sure and don't like (or similar concept language), to express their thoughts and feelings around the given topic. This then allows the learner to participate in conversations and decision-making processes more effectively. This innovative tool fosters inclusive and accessible communication, making it especially valuable in healthcare, education and social care settings, where it empowers all individuals to have a voice and be actively involved in their own lives and care.

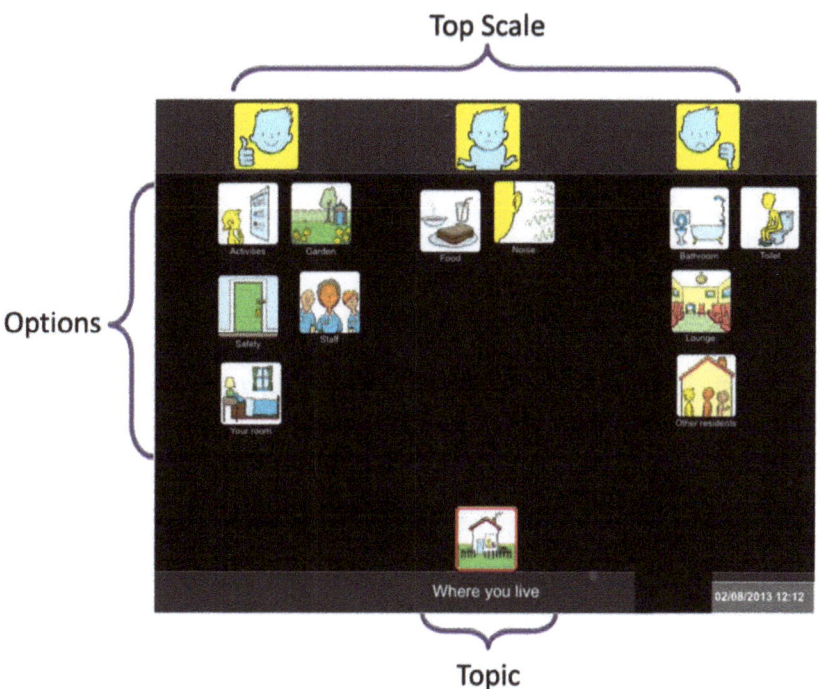

Figure 15.5 This image shows a black image with symbols.

Source: The symbols are designed and © to Adam Murphy 2015 and assigned to Talking Mats Ltd. in perpetuity. They may not be reproduced without permission. www.talkingmats.com

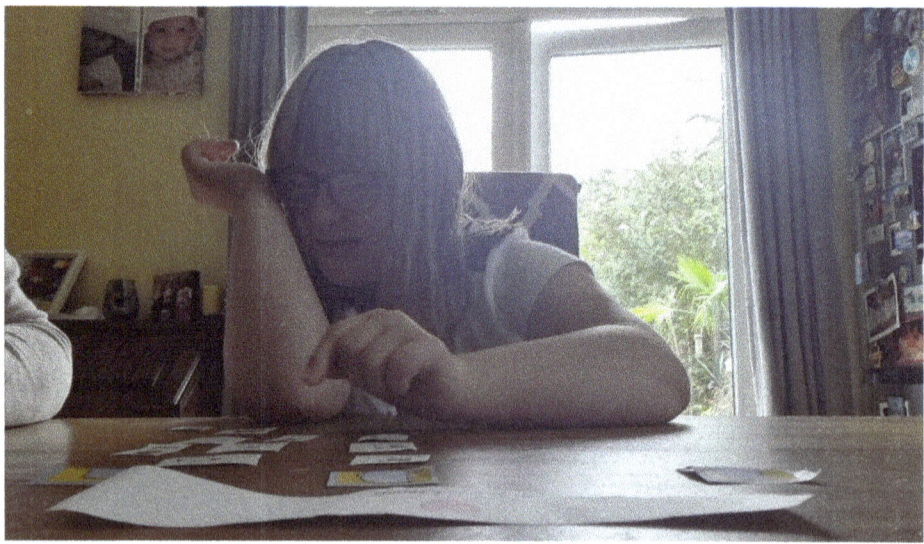

Figure 15.6 This image shows a girl pointing to symbols.

Source: Photographed by the author, used with permission.

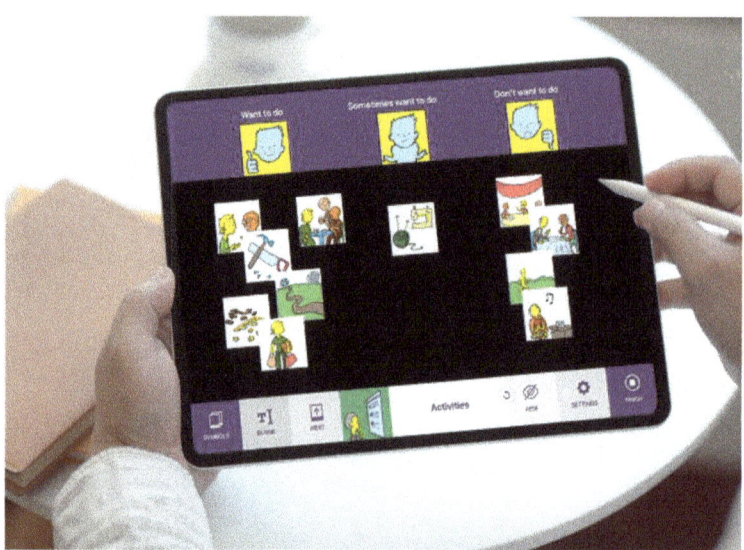

Figure 15.7 This image shows a black image with symbols and a hand.

Source: The symbols are designed and © to Adam Murphy 2015 and assigned to Talking Mats Ltd. in perpetuity. They may not be reproduced without permission. www.talkingmats.com

To use a Talking Mat, a facilitator or communicator presents the mat to the learner. When presented with a symbol by the communication partner, the learner can then use their hand, fist or eye point to indicate where they want to put the symbol on the mat, anywhere along the scale of the thumbs up, unsure or thumbs down symbols.

Figure 15.6 was a Talking Mat which was completed by Emmy in lockdown for her to express her opinions about school activities ahead of her EHCP review meeting. As it was during lockdown, some elements had to be improvised, for example, using a clear surface instead of a mat to place the symbols on.

Talking Mats is also available in app form for learners who may be more familiar and comfortable with accessing the resource digitally via a touch screen (Figure 15.7).

Talking Mats is a good tool to promote authentic pupil voice in school council meetings.

The goals of school councils are to empower learners and promote pupil voice in the school and for the representatives to have the opportunity to represent their peers and be the voice for change in their school. By using tools such as Talking Mats and aided language displays more learners can share their thoughts and opinions on matters addressed. Talking Mats have a range of training available to support your skill development in this area.

The Real-life Impact of Fostering Pupil Voice

Once learners understand that they have a voice and they will be listened to, it can have a massive impact on all aspects of their life.

Safeguarding

By teaching learners how to communicate and showing them that their thoughts and opinions will be listened to and given due weight, we are also giving them a tool to protect themselves.

Safeguarding concerns for children who cannot use verbal speech require particularly careful attention, as their communication barriers can make it challenging for them to express their needs, feelings, or report any potential harm or abuse. Giving children the confidence, as well as the aided language/AAC to speak out could be life changing for them.

Medical Appointments

Aided language/AAC can also be highly effective in enhancing the quality of medical appointments for learners with SLCN. By providing these children with a means to express their needs, symptoms, and concerns, aided language/AAC can bridge the communication gap, ensuring their voices are heard in the healthcare setting. Whether through picture boards, AAC devices, or sign language, AAC allows non-verbal children to actively participate in their medical care, providing critical information to healthcare professionals for accurate diagnosis and treatment.

Using rating scales like the one shown earlier, and body chart aided language displays (Figure 15.8) can be a very effective way for a child to participate in their appointment. Using aided language/AAC promotes a sense of empowerment and reduces anxiety during medical appointments which can create a more positive experience for the child who may already be anxious in the unfamiliar context.

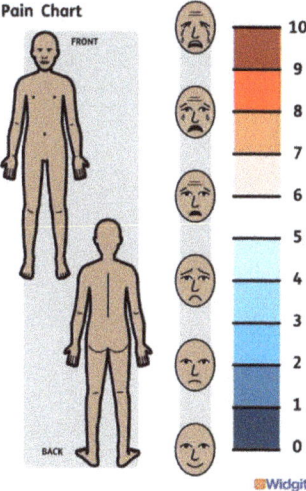

Figure 15.8 This image shows a body and coloured scale.
Source: Widgit Symbols © Widgit Software Ltd 2002–2023. www.widgit.com

Taking their Place in Society

When we think about using AAC and aided language to promote pupil voice, then the end goal, is of course, that the learner grows up to take their place in society. To have control over their own lives and where possible to contribute to society. That may be by gaining a job, voting or contributing to general family life.

By teaching a learner how to express themselves using aided language/AAC and then showing them that their voice will be listened to, is one of the most powerful things we can teach a learner with significant SLCN.

Conclusion

This chapter has looked at a selection of tools to support your classroom practice to elicit pupil voice from your learners with Speech, Language and Communication Needs. It has demonstrated how having aided language resources available in the school environment can facilitate the learner to more readily share their thoughts and opinions on a day-to-day level. Tools such as Talking Mats help learners to understand that their opinions are welcomed and provide you with information on which you can act, to show the learner their opinions are being given due weight.

In order to ensure that pupil voice is heard and given due weight, it is key that a whole school approach is taken. The next chapter looks at how you can promote the use of aided language/AAC consistently throughout your school by tackling organisational change by the introduction of an AAC policy.

Bibliography

Department for Education and Department of Health (2015). Special Educational Needs and Disability Code of Practice: 0 to 25 years. Ref: DFE-00205-2013 Available at: www.gov.uk/government/publications/send-code-of-practice-0-to-25

Department for Education and Department of Health (2022). SEND Review: Right support Right place Right time. Available at: https://assets.publishing.service.gov.uk/media/624178c68fa8f5277c0168e7/SEND_review_right_support_right_place_right_time_accessible.pdf

Mats, T. (2013). What is a Talking Mat? – Improving Communication, Improving Lives. [online] Talking Mats. Available at: www.talkingmats.com/about/what-is-a-talking-mat/

Sharma, P. (2021). Barriers Faced When Eliciting the Voice of Children and Young People With Special Educational Needs and Disabilities for their Education, Health and Care Plans and Annual Reviews. *British Journal of Special Education*, 48(4), 455–476. doi: https://doi.org/10.1111/1467-8578.12386

16 Whole School Approach to Supporting Learners with Speech, Language and Communication Needs

This chapter considers the importance of a whole school approach to supporting learners who use aided language/AAC. Before discussing why a whole school approach is needed, it is worthwhile looking back to the evidence base and understanding why supporting learners with AAC systems is often unsuccessful.

Thinking back to Chapter eight and the research of Johnson et al. (2006) around device abandonment, key themes were identified around time, training, transition and staff confidence, all of which could be addressed at organisational level.

Having a strong structure and ethos in place across the educational setting, many of the factors identified by Johnson et al. can be negated. This makes it sound a simple task, however, in reality we know that organisational change takes time and can be challenging.

An effective way to begin the journey of organisational change to support AAC learners within your setting is to create an AAC policy. This may sit as a stand-alone policy, or within the school's existing communication policy.

Policy documents can often sit unread on a school server and website and have no perceived worth. At best, the majority of the staff team have read it and may have had some input. The worst case scenario is that it is a document that has been copied and pasted from another organisation and edited to be personalised to the school.

For true organisational change the document must be created in a collaborative way with key stakeholders from across the setting. These stakeholders form a working party and should have representatives such as:

- A member of the senior leadership team: This person's role is to liaise between the working party and the senior leadership team, to ensure that what is suggested in the policy document is able to be honoured throughout day-to-day practice. What the working party would like to happen and what the school is able to deliver, due to financial or staffing constraints, may be two different things. The member of the senior leadership team in the working party will take on the role of negotiator with the wider senior leadership team.
- Speech and language therapist: Not all education settings will have access to a speech and language therapist but, if your setting does, then please think to include them in the co-production of the AAC policy. Remember, education is not an island, and working in a multidisciplinary manner helps to establish things like appropriate onward referral pathways to access NHS-funded AAC, where appropriate.
- The school's communication lead: This person is likely to be the go-to for anything communication related in the school. They will be the one who is likely to have attended external training sessions around AAC and aided language and has a whole-school oversight on current practice.
- Classroom practitioners: These individuals are the people in classrooms. They may be teachers or teaching assistants. They are at the frontline of delivery. The roles of these people on the working party are to give feedback to the rest of the team around realistic expectations on the wider staff team in implementing the AAC policy.

When co creating an AAC policy it may be useful to use a template as a guide to support discussion, ensuring that your working party discusses all angles that need to be covered.

Ace Centre have produced a free AAC policy guide which a working party could use to facilitate their discussions whilst creating that personalised policy (Figure 16.1).

Ace Centre created the guidance document in 2024 whilst working with a selection of specialist schools. They supported schools in the co-production of the schools' AAC policy, and the guidance document reflects some of the feedback and discussions from the various working parties within those schools.

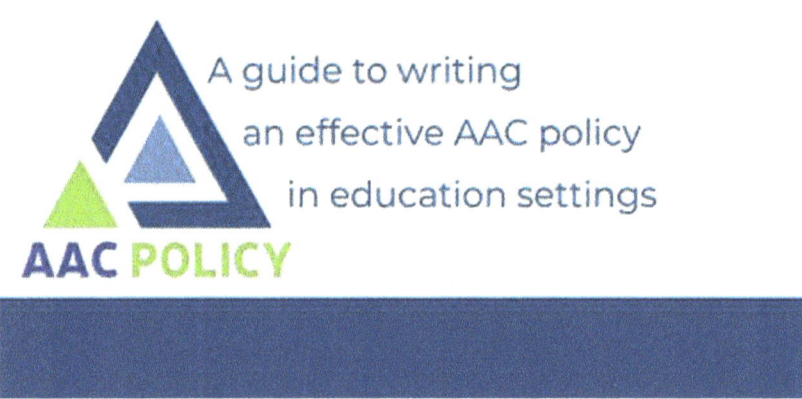

Figure 16.1 This image shows the logo for the Ace Centre's guidance document on writing an AAC policy.
Source: Created by Ace Centre. https://acecentre.org.uk/resources

Some key themes identified to be discussed and reflected in the creation of an AAC policy are:

- The school's vision/aims
- Terminology explained
- Current legislation
- The current educational context
- Roles and responsibilities – which then links to training and referral pathways
- Funding options

Giving clarification around these key areas will help to facilitate organisational change. It would be worthwhile here to go into greater detail around these identified areas.

The School's Vision/Aims

Most school policies start with giving the current context of the school/college. How many learners attend, what are the needs of the cohort of learners, what the school/college aims to achieve with the policy.

Brays School in Birmingham gathered the whole school staff together and collaboratively created a pledge (Figure 16.2).

Terminology Explained

As discussed in a previous chapter, schools can be terminology heavy, and the working party must keep at the forefront of their minds who the policy is for. The policy document needs to be accessible for all stakeholders, such as families, new staff and existing staff to read and understand. Thinking about what terminology is used within your educational setting and documenting this promotes a shared understanding and a common language when driving that organisational change. There is no point having an AAC policy that readers do not understand. That will just promote disengagement from the stakeholders and will act as a barrier to change.

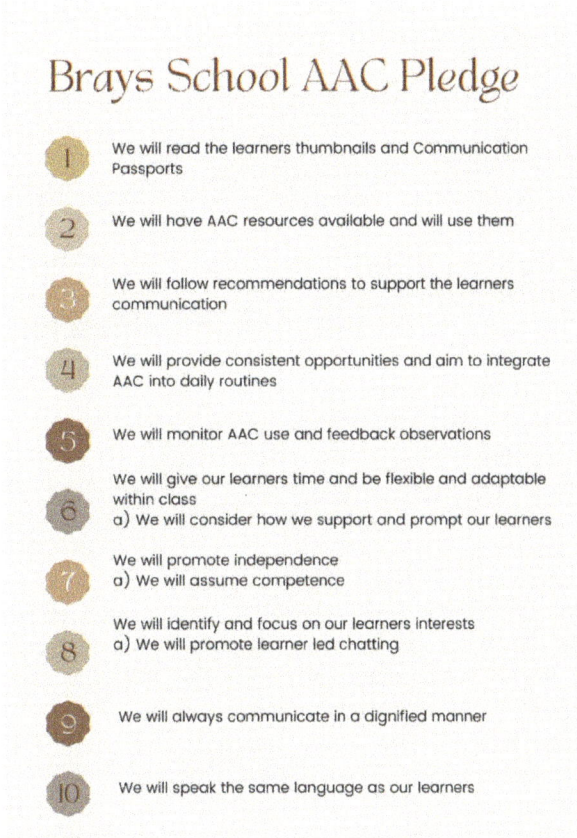

Figure 16.2 This image shows a list of 10 points.

Source: With thanks to Brays School for sharing this pledge.

The Current Legislation

The working party driving the organisational change to support the use of aided language and AAC in the educational setting, should also read and document key legislation around facilitating the use of aided language. This legislation is shared in one of the earlier chapters. In Ace Centre's Policy guidance document, they highlighted that the majority of working parties they worked with were not aware of the current legislation. The legislation helps readers of the policy to understand the importance of facilitating communication using aided language for their learners.

The Current Educational Context

The Department for Education also refer heavily to ensuring that learners have a voice, and that voice is heard. They advocate that learners should express opinions about their lives and communicate choices in decisions that affect them. This is often referred to as pupil voice within school settings. Pupil voice has been discussed in the previous chapter. Referencing the SEND Code of Practice 2015 in policy highlights the standards expected from the Department for Education in schools. This section and the section on legislation raise the status of the policy to the likes of other policies covered in legislation, such as the health and safety policy.

Roles and Responsibilities

This section forms the meatiest area for discussion for any working party creating an AAC policy. It may be useful here to share a case example from Brays School in Birmingham.

Case Example – Brays School in Birmingham

Brays School began with the team auditing current aided language/AAC in general classroom practice at the school (Figure 16.3). They identified things such as aided language modelling, Objects of Reference, Makaton, visual timetables, PECS, AAC apps on iPads, Communication Books, Tassles and key words (aided language displays).

This information was noted down in one of the working party's meetings.

Then the working party identified what they expected all staff to know. This information sat at the bottom tier of their pyramid.

The next tier up they identified as themselves. The working party were the group of people who would take responsibility for driving organisational change. Therefore, they identified that they would need to know how to implement all of the AAC within tier one. On top of that, they would also need to be competent in delivering training and support around the AAC listed in tier two of their pyramid. Tier three of their pyramid related to onward referrals for AAC from external agencies, such as the local NHS Speech and Language Therapy Team and the NHS England Specialised Service for AAC Users.

After the initial discussion was recorded on paper, a diagram of this current provision was created. This image was then included in Brays' AAC policy, as a clear visual aid to all on the different referral processes. Brays School identified that all staff should be able to identify that there was either a need for a personalised AAC system or that there was an issue with a learner's current AAC system and they should know who to go to for support on the communication team. The communication team then know when it's appropriate to refer to the local NHS speech and language therapy team. Then the local NHS therapist will make any appropriate referrals to the NHS England Specialised Service for AAC users with supporting information provided by the communication team.

Having a visual to explain the onward referral process made it clear who is responsible for making which referrals.

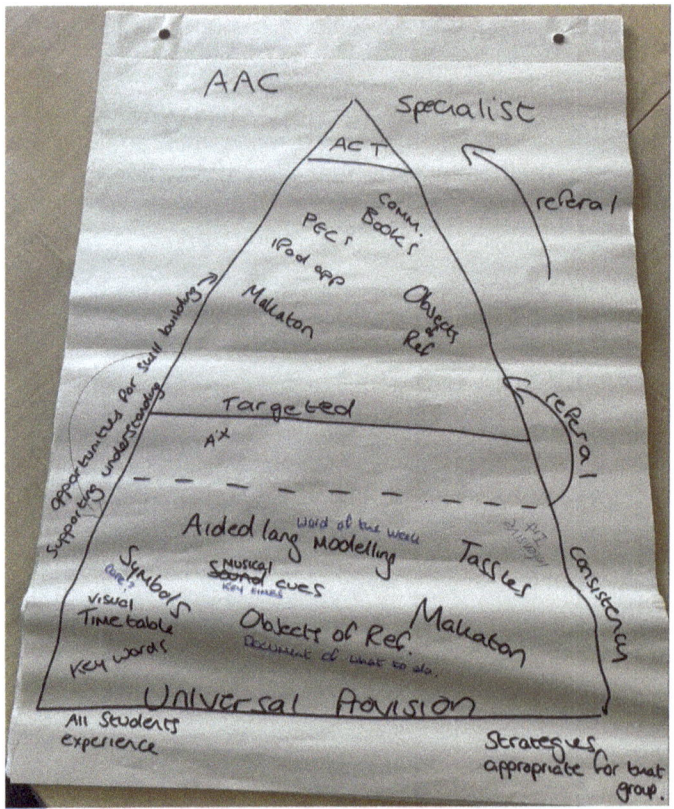

Figure 16.3 Image shows a hand drawn flip chart page of a tiered pyramid.

Source: Photographed by the author.

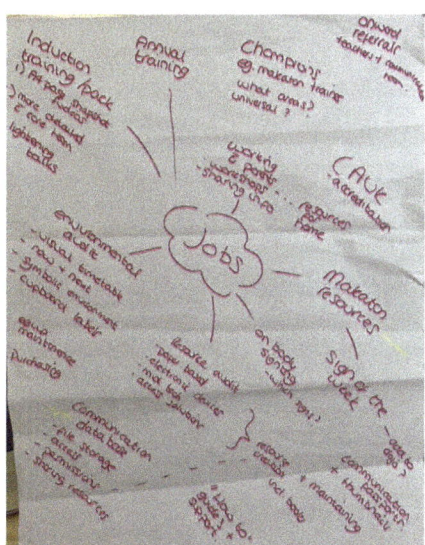

Figure 16.4 Image shows a handwritten mind map.

Source: Photographed by the author.

Identifying Responsibilities for the Core Team Driving Organisational Change

Going through this process allowed the team members to identify that they would each need to hold different roles and responsibilities within the team. For example, one person may need to be responsible for training all staff to use the symbol generating software, such as Boardmaker software, so the wider team are easily able to make aided language displays for their classrooms. The working party recorded all the 'jobs' that going through the process of establishing roles and responsibilities had highlighted (Figure 16.4).

Training

Identifying roles and responsibilities inevitably led to discussions around training for staff at all levels of the pyramid. Although training needs do not always have to be included in the outward-facing policy, the identification and recording training needs should sit alongside the policy and be the action plan for the first steps in driving organisational change.

Before identifying what level of training was required for staff in different roles across the school, it was important to benchmark the staff's current skill set. To do this Brays School used a self-audit tool from NHS Scotland called IPAACKS – Informing and Profiling Augmentative and Alternative Communication (AAC) Knowledge and Skills.

"The Scottish Government published the report, A Right to Speak: Supporting Individuals who use Augmentative and Alternative Communication in June 2012. The report's recommendations included the need to ensure that people who use AAC (augmentative and alternative communication) have access to appropriate levels of high-quality specialist assessment and support delivered as locally as possible. NHS Education for Scotland (NES) developed IPAACKS to improve the experiences, opportunities and quality of life of people who use AAC by ensuring that the people who work with them have the knowledge, skills and values required for their roles. Different members of the workforce may require specific knowledge and skills depending on their role." www.aacscotland.org.uk/files/cm/files/ipaacks.pdf

IPAACKS highlights competencies in eight areas. These areas are:

- Identification of Need
- Assessment
- Implementation
- Review
- Technology: preparation, adaptation, integration
- Technology: management of resources
- AAC Leadership
- Facilitating Learning

The tool itself has a range of statements over four levels for each of the eight areas. Staff read the different statements and profiled themselves against them according to which level best suits their current knowledge and skill levels. Once the staff member has profiled themselves, the IPAACKS tool allows them to create a pie chart of their skills across the eight areas.

These are case examples from staff who hold different roles within Brays School who completed the IPAACKS self-audit tool.

Universal Tier Level Staff Member

When the team at Brays School profiled themselves, they identified that the universal level of staff (the wider staff team) had a solid level one across six of the areas. They profiled themselves at level two for identifying need and review. These are the staff in the classrooms, working with the learner's day to day.

Communication Team Staff Member

When the communication team profiled their skills around AAC, they identified with level two in most of the eight areas. The exceptions were level three in 'Identifying Need and Review', so a similar increase in skills in those areas was seen, as with the rest of the wider staff team, who also identified themselves as higher in this area. However, they identified as level one for Technology: Management of Resources.

Communication Lead

The communication lead in the school identified a higher skill level, sitting at level three for almost all the eight categories. This was a member of staff who had been identified to drive the communication group and the main person in the school with a responsibility around communication support.

Assistive Technologist: IT Speciality

When the working party began the roles and responsibilities section of their policy, they identified a role which was quite separate from the rest of the team. That was the role of an assistive technologist. They identified the need for a person who had the technical skills to problem-solve the technology when the wider team identified problems with it. This person did not need high level skills across all areas but did need high level skills in using, and problem-solving, technology. This could be to support users with electronic AAC or users who require assistive technology to access their AAC, such as a learner using an eye gaze camera to control the AAC.

Once skills were audited, the Brays team were able to identify what training was required and what training they would be responsible for delivering. They made an action plan of training, which needed to be delivered annually to the team working within the universal staff tier. They also planned out what training would need to be delivered within the staff induction program.

The training programs they identified and built into the school's continual professional development program were the driving force for organisational change.

Funding

One of the last sections Ace Centre identified in their policy guidance document was funding. When creating their policy document, Brays School began to explore funding streams to provide electronic AAC for learners who voice output AAC was most appropriate for them. When Bray began its journey, the school felt it was their responsibility to fund electronic AAC for some learners. This was problematic as the school felt unsure of what would be most appropriate AAC to purchase to meet the individual needs of the learners. Once working through their policy document there became a shared understanding of NHS referral pathways for AAC in their area.

The working party reached out to the local NHS therapy team and were able to establish referral pathways for support, even though the national shortage of NHS therapists was

> also evident in their area at the time the policy was being created. Working in a multidisciplinary way with the NHS, Speech and Language Therapists allowed funding options to be explored jointly.
>
> A full copy of the Brays School AAC Policy Document can be downloaded by following the access instructions at the front of this book. With thanks to Brays School.

Typically, most AAC needs are met by the local speech and language therapy teams. In reality however, this is not a commissioned service, and local teams often do not have access to a pot of money to fund this, which can be very frustrating to everyone involved. The picture varies nationally from area to area. In some areas education and health combine funding for those 90 per cent of AAC users who do not meet the criteria for the NHS England Specialised Service for AAC pathway. If you find yourself in a position where an assessment has identified the need for electronic AAC, and there is no NHS funding, then there are a small selection of charities who currently fund AAC devices. Smartbox have a range of charities displayed on their webpage. https://thinksmartbox.com/funding/funding-uk/

There are currently 17 NHS England Specialised Service for AAC Hubs. The services the hubs offer vary from assessments and provision of equipment, short-term loans of equipment and training.

The NHS hubs are commissioned to assess 10 per cent of the population with the most complex AAC needs. You can find out more about your local hub from the information below. If you are unsure who your local hub is you can find out on the Service Finder tool on the Ace Centre website. https://acecentre.org.uk/nhs-service-finder

Conclusion

Every policy should be personalised to each educational setting. That is how organisational change happens. It is by identifying the uniqueness of the educational setting, as well as the individuals supported in that setting, and taking steps to plan the journey to where you want to be as a school supporting AAC users.

Bibliography

IPAACKS Informing and Profiling Augmentative and Alternative Communication (AAC) Knowledge and Skills Supporting the learning and development of people working with individuals who use AAC enter. (n.d.). Available at: www.aacscotland.org.uk/files/cm/files/ipaacks.pdf

Johnson, J.M., Inglebret, E., Jones, C. and Ray, J. (2006). Perspectives of Speech Language Pathologists Regarding Success Versus Abandonment of AAC. *Augmentative and Alternative Communication*, 22(2), pp.85–99. doi: https://doi.org/10.1080/07434610500483588

17 Final Thoughts

Keywords: Whole School Ethos; Aided Language; Augmentative and Alternative Communication (AAC); Staff Training; Implementation Strategies; Modelling; Speech, Language and Communication Needs (SLCN)

This book has had a deep dive into how you can change classroom and whole school practice around the implementation of aided language/AAC for learners with Speech, Language and Communication Needs (SLCN). If you embark on this journey to leave a legacy of good practice, which is embedded into the ethos of the school, then policy is paramount. Creating an AAC policy with key stakeholders will give you a strong foundation on which to build effective classroom practice for those learners, ensuring that staff are trained and confident in how to support them.

Introducing aided language/AAC can be daunting, especially if you have limited access to a speech and language therapist for guidance. Please do not panic, the research has shown us that introducing aided language does not hinder the development of verbal speech. The terminology around aided language/AAC may feel overwhelming, but as with everything else in life, strip it back and you'll realise that we are just talking about the learner being able to chat with other people.

For learners to develop their language, modelling is key. Learners will not make progress without being shown how to use aided language/AAC. Using the learner's AAC system will enable them to see a model of how to use this effectively. It's a language development journey for some learners using aided language/AAC, so goal setting keeps that journey moving forward. Having a good understanding and overview of the current stage of your learner's language development and the next steps, will support you in ensuring learners are not treading water. Remember, breaking goals down into smaller chunks allows the learner to experience success, as they are more achievable.

When a learner is unable to point to symbols, it does not mean they cannot use aided language to communicate. For learners with the most complex physical disabilities, it may appear that they do not have the cognitive ability to use aided language/AAC. However, consider how a learner's world may be unlocked by looking at alternative ways to access resources. A physical disability should never be viewed as a barrier to communication.

The book stresses the importance of autonomous communication. Whether we call it pupil voice or just communication, the end goal is the same. We want our learners with SLCN to be confident in expressing themselves and to take their place in society. Introducing the use of aided language can facilitate this for those learners who are not yet literate.

Technology is constantly evolving and who knows how it may be able to facilitate our learners with Speech, Language and Communication Needs in the future, but remember, the goal here is access to language. Technology is not always the key to unlocking the door.

Index

Note: Page numbers in *italics* indicate figures.

AAC *see* Augmentative and Alternative Communication
AAC Bootcamp 85
AAC policy 2, 181–182, 187; case example 184–187, *184–185*; current educational context 183; current legislation 183; guide 181, *182*, 183, 186; roles and responsibilities 183–187, *184–185*; school's vision/aims 182, *183*; stakeholders 181; terminology 182
AAC prompt hierarchy 67, *68*, 123–127, *125–126*
ACA (Affective Communication Assessment) 67, *98*, 96–101, *100*
access wobble switches 144, *144*
Ace Centre: AAC policy guide 181, *182*, 183, 186; communication boards *11*, 110; communication books 107–108; core and fringe vocabulary *17*, 17; eye-pointing resources 113, 114–115, *115*; financial guidance 41; Look2Talk book 152, *153*; Pragmatic Profile 93, 96; Service finder tool 187; Simon Says symbol chart *153*; *Speakbook* 115; spelling charts 117, *117*; support 40; symbol sets 59
Affective Communication Assessment (ACA) 69, *98*, 96–101, *100*
aided communication 10
aided language 10, 189; abandonment 42–3; assessment and target setting 163–170; common types of SCLN needs 38; communication partners 119–125, 133, 135; confusion around terminology 39; core and fringe vocabulary 17; currently used strategies 39–40, *39–40*; environment 47–59; financial barriers 41; language development 91–93, 96, 99; meaning of 39, 59; modelling 77–78, 83, 85, 88; multidisciplinary team 42; myths and misconceptions 19–26; organisational barriers 41–42, *41*; paper-based resources 103, 118; physical disabilities, learners with 137–139, 143, 150, 152, 160; pupil voice 175, 179–180; symbols 59–64; teaching symbolic language 65–74; training 38–43; whole school approach 181–187
Aided Language Displays (ALDs) 48–49, *49–50*; context-specific 50–52, *51–52*; large-scale 52–54, *54*; medical appointments 179; physical disabilities, learners with 137, 142; pupil voice 175, *176–177*, 178, 179; small-scale 55, *56*; teaching symbolic language 65; toilet aided language display *51*
aided language simulation/input *see* modelling
aims, school's 182, *183*
ALDs *see* aided language displays
alphabet charts 117–118, *117*

alternative access 13, 42; *see also* physical disabilities, learners with
alternative mice 155–160, *155–160*
annual reviews 174, 175, 178
Applied Behaviour Analysis (ABA) 93
apron with symbols 55–56, *55*
assessment and target setting 163–164, 170; Communication Matrix 165–170, *169*; Dynamic AAC Goals Grid-3 164–165; joint 27–28; *see also* target reviews
Assistive Technology (ATech): AAC policy 186; eye pointing 151; scanning 142; technical barriers 42; *see also* electronic AAC
AssistiveWare: Affective Communication Assessment 99; communication boards 112; Do's and Don'ts of AAC poster 85, *86*; teaching symbolic language 69, *70*; training and support 40
Augmentative and Alternative Communication (AAC) 189; abandonment 37–38, 42–43, 123, 181; assessment and target setting 163–170; commonly used 10–13, *10–13*; communication partners 17, 119–125, 133–135; confusion around terminology 39; core and fringe vocabulary 17, 18; currently used strategies 39–40, *39–40*; financial barriers to implementation of 40–41; forcing 82–83; language development 93–102; legislation 2; meaning of 10, 39; modelling 77–88; multidisciplinary team 42; myths and misconceptions 19–26; organisational barriers 41–42, *41*; paper-based resources 103–104, 117–118; physical disabilities, learners with 139, 160; pupil voice 179–180; success factors 43; symbols 60, 62, 64; teaching symbolic language 65–74; technical barriers 42; training 38–43; unaided versus aided 10; *see also* AAC policy; AAC prompt hierarchy; electronic AAC
autism: aided language displays 55; applied behaviour analysis 93; PECS 91, 93
autonomous voice *see* pupil voice

babbling 70–71
ball stylus *140*
Blue2 switches 145
Bluetooth: joysticks 157; switches 145, *147*; trackballs 156
Boardmaker 45, 64, 103, 105; eye-pointing resources 114
Boardmaker symbols *see* PCS symbols
Brays School, Birmingham: pledge 182, *183*; roles and responsibilities 183–187, *184–185*
Bryan, Johnathan 113
Burkhart, Linda 61

Index

Call Scotland 40
cars aided language display 50–1, *51*
Center for Literacy and Disability Studies: communication boards 110; eye-pointing resources 114, *114*; Project Core Implementation Model 137; Universal Core Selection Tool 137
cerebral palsy 137
charities 187
choice boards 23, 55, *54*; breaktime 92; language development 91–92
Clicker 64
closed questions 132–133
coaching communication partners 135
cognitive development, Piaget's stages of 21–22; Affective Communication Assessment 93–94, *99*
collaborative working *see* multidisciplinary team; teamwork
Communicate in Print 48, 103, 105; eye-pointing resources 114
Communication Access UK 121
Communication Bill of Rights 4; examples *4–5*
communication boards *11*, 12; library of resources 110–114; modelling 77
communication books *3*, *12*, 12; case example 2; duplicates 103; eye-pointing 114, *115*; library of resources 107–109; terminology 13–15
communication breakdowns 19; communication partners 122–123; Pragmatic Profile 96
communication charts *see* aided language displays
Communication Matrix 165–170, *169*; support 40
communication partners 6, 17, *18*, 135; AAC device abandonment 37; AAC prompt hierarchy 123–127, *125–126*; aided language displays 48, 52; autonomy, importance of 127–129, *129*; characteristics of 121–122, *121–122*; choice boards 55; coaching 135; communication breakdowns 122–123; Communication Matrix 166–168; communicative competencies 74–75; directive versus non-directive language 129–133, *132*; environment 48; importance of 121; language development 41, 91, 96; means, reasons and opportunities 133–135, *133*; modelling 77–86, 88; myths and misconceptions 19, 21, 23; paper-based resources 103–104, 113, 118; people classed as 119, *119*; physical disabilities, learners with 137, 142–143, 151–152; PODD 101; problems with hand-over-hand prompting 127, *128*; pupil voice 177–178; what they will benefit from 119–120
communication passports 19; Affective Communication Assessment 99; benefits 31–34; teamwork 30–34, *32–33*
communication turns table 131–132, *132*
communicative competencies: Dynamic AAC Goals Grid-3 (DAGG) 164; teaching symbolic language 71–72
communicative functions: assessment and target setting 164; language development 91–93, *95*, 96–97, *97–98*, 100–101, *101*
compliance versus autonomy 127–129, *129*
Convention on the Rights of Persons with Disabilities (CPRD) 2
Convention on the Rights of the Child 2, 173
core vocabulary 15, *15*, 17, 25; aided language displays 48, 51; Communication Matrix 167; modelling 78, 79, 83; PODD 100; teaching symbolic language 70, *70–71*

Dear Zoo 48–49, *49–50*
delivery of speech and language therapy 39
Department for Education (DfE): AAC policy 183; documentation 164; *see also* SEN Code of Practice; SEND review
descriptive teaching 79
Devereux, Kathleen 61
directive language 129–132
Dynamic AAC Goals Grid-3 164–165
dynamic displays 14

Early Years settings: aided language displays 49; apron with symbols 55–56; environment 48
EasyChat 87–88
Education, Health and Care Plans (EHCPs) 3; assessment and target setting 164; pupil voice 175, *176*, 178; SEND review 4, 38; teamwork 29–30
electronic AAC *12–13*, 12–13; AAC policy 186; affordability 22; drawbacks 103, 113; environment 55–56; financial barriers 40–41; modelling 78, 82, 83; natural language development 21; organisational barriers 42; physical disabilities, learners with 137–160; pupil voice 178; Talking Mats 178, *178*; teaching symbolic language 70–72; technical barriers 42; terminology 13–15; training 40
Engagement Scale Model 165
environment 48–48, *45–47*, 57; aided language displays (ALDs) 48–49, *49–50*; apron with symbols 56, *56*; choice boards *54*, 55; context-specific ALDs 50–52, *51*; electronic AAC 56; eye gaze technology 155; large-scale ALDs 52–54, *53*; small-scale ALDs 53, *56*
equipment requirements, visual support *46*
E-Tran frames 113, *113–114*, 113, 152
expressive language 9; Affective Communication Assessment 99; communication passports 34; environment 45, 48–57; myths and misconceptions 19–20, 23; symbol sets 59; teaching symbolic language 67, 69
eye gaze *see* eye pointing/gaze
Eye Gaze Learning Curve 154
eye-link 115, *116*
eye pointing/gaze 153–155, *154*; paper-based resources 113–115, *113–116*, 117; physical disabilities, learners with 151–153, *153–154*; spelling charts 117

fatigue, and eye gaze technology 154
financial barriers 40–41; AAC policy 186–187
Fitzgerald key 106
freedom of speech 1
fringe vocabulary 16–17, *17*, 25; aided language displays 48, 52–54; teaching symbolic language 69, *70*

goal setting *see* assessment and target setting
GoTalk *13*
graphic symbols 59–64; hierarchy of symbolic understanding 23, *25*; teaching 65–74; 'you' 60
group modelling 83
The Gruffalo 125, *125*

hand-over-hand prompting 126–127; problems with 124, *128*
happy accidents 71
head mice 158, *158*
hierarchy of symbolic understanding 23, *25*, *94*
high contrast symbols 59; PCS 61, *62*
human rights 1, 3
hybrid displays 14

immunisations, visual schedule for *45*
Inclusive Technology: Eye Gaze Learning Curve 154; Switch Progression Road Map *147*, 148; switch skill development 150
inclusivity: aided language displays 51, 54; PCS high contrast symbols 61
integrated joysticks 157
integrated therapy: reviews 29; teamwork 28, *29*, 29
interaction characteristics 122
International Society for Augmentative and Alternative Communication 10
interventions, and teamwork 28, *29*
IPAACKS 185–186
iSwitches 145, *147*

Jelly Bean switches 144, *145*
Johnson, Roxie 60
Joyce, Patrick 115
joysticks 157, *157*

keyguards 141, *141*
keyrings 55
Key Stage One 50

language development *23*, 23, 67, 91–93, 101; Affective Communication Assessment *98*, 96–98, *101*; babbling 70–71; communication partners 41, 121, 125; hierarchy of symbolic understanding 23; paper-based resources 104, 118; physical disabilities, learners with 137; profiling tools 93–96, *97–98*
language functions *see* communicative functions
lanyards 55, *55*
'last resort' myth 20
legislation, and AAC policy 183
Liberator: communication boards 111; communication books 108; Easy Chat 51, 52, *53*; lanyard 55; symbol sets 59; teaching symbolic language 70, *72–73*; training and support 40; WordPower vocabulary 83, *84*
Look 2 Talk books 108, 114, *115*, 152, *153*

medical appointments 179, *179*
mental health 1; waiting for natural speech to develop 20
mice alternatives 155–160, *155–160*
mice settings 158–160, *158–160*
Microsoft Learning Tools: Immersive Reader 64; PCS symbols 64
modelling 77, 88, 189; Affective Communication Assessment 99; aided language displays 48–49; apron with symbols 55–56; to attribute meaning 80–81; beginning 77–78; benefits 69; descriptive teaching 79; electronic AAC 55; forcing versus 82–83; group 83; importance 69; multidisciplinary team 42; myths and misconceptions 21; nature of 77; personal 79–80, *80*; pupil voice 175; scaffolding 81–82, *81–82*; structured lessons versus 85; teaching symbolic language 69; tips 83–84, *84*, *86*; *see also* peer modelling
mouldable strap stylus *140*
mouse alternatives 155–160, *155–160*
mouse settings 158–160, *158–160*
multidisciplinary team 39, 42; AAC policy 181, 186; assessment and target setting 163; language development 91, 93; physical disabilities, learners with 146, 150; *see also* teamwork
multiple message devices *13*, 13

National Curriculum 164
National Health Service (NHS) 41, 184–187
natural speech 20–21, *21*
non-directive language 129–133
NovaChats 83
now and next board *47*

objects of reference 10, *10*; hierarchy of symbolic understanding 23
open questions 132–133
organisational barriers 41–42, *41*

Pace Centre 149–150, *150*
page sets 14
Pal Pad switches 144–145, *146*
paper-based resources 118; accessing 106; alphabet/spelling charts 117–118, *117*; attributes 103; barriers to implementing 104; considerations for creating 105; downloadable 114–115, *115–116*; eye pointing 113–115, *113–116*, 152, *153*, 154; library of 107–112; organisation of 106; personalisation 105, 118; physical disabilities, learners with 137, 152, *153*, 154; positives 103–104; skills developed by use of 104; symbol sets 105–106
partner assisted scanning 142–143, *142–143*, 154; spelling charts 117
PCS symbols *14*, 14, 60, *61*, 64, 105; high-contrast 61, *62*
PECS (Picture Exchange Communication System) *11*, 11, *92*; hand-over-hand prompting 127; language development 91–93
peer modelling 87, 88; case study 87–88, *87–88*; electronic AAC 56–57; teamwork 28
personalisation: paper-based resources 105, 118; spelling charts 118
personal modelling 79–80, *80*; teaching symbolic language 66
physical disabilities, learners with 137, 156, 189; alternative mice 155–160, *155–160*; eye pointing 151–155, *153–154*; scanning 142–146, *142–147*; switch skill development 146–150, *147*, *150–152*; touch access 137–141, *138–141*
Piaget's stages of cognitive development 21–22; Affective Communication Assessment *99*, 97
Picture Communication Symbols (PCS) *see* PCS symbols
Picture Exchange Communication System *see* PECS
pillow switches 145, *146*
PODD (Pragmatic Organisation of Dramatic Displays) 61, 107; communication books *12*; language development 100–101, *101*

point talking *see* modelling
policy *see* AAC policy
Porter, Gayle 61, 107
pragmatic language *23*, 93–96, *95*, 101
Pragmatic Organisation of Dramatic Displays *see* PODD
Pragmatic Profile 68–69, 93–97, *97–98*
primary education 48
profiling tools 93–96, *97–98*
Project Core 15, *16*; communication boards 110; eye-pointing resources 114
ProloQuo 112
ProloQuo2Go *13*, *14*, 14, 112; core word board *81*, 82
prompting 78; *see also* AAC prompt hierarchy
pupil voice 1, 173–174, 180, 189; AAC policy 183; aided language displays 175, *176–177*; barriers to 174–175, *174*; importance of 124–129, *129*; legislation 4; medical appointments 179, *179*; safeguarding 179; SEN Code of Practice 3; society, place in 179–180; Talking Mats 177–178, *177–178*

Rebus symbols *see* Widgit symbols
receptive language 9; communication passports 34; environment 45, 55; language development 91; symbol sets 59
referential teaching 79
rollerballs 156, *156*
Royal College of Speech and Language Therapists: Clinical Information on Mental Health (adults) 1; Communication Access UK 121; Speech Language and Communication Needs, meaning of 9

safeguarding: aided language displays 51; pupil voice 179
scaffolding 66, 81–82, *81–82*
scanning 143–146, *142–147*, 154; patterns (switch skill development) 150, *151–152*
school councils 178
school routine, visual support *47*
secondary education 48
SEN Code of Practice 3, 9; AAC policy 183; Education, Health and Care Plans 29–30; pupil voice 173
SEND review 4, 38; pupil voice 173
SEN Support 4
Seven Stages of Switch Development 149–150, *150*
Simon Says symbol chart *153*
single message devices *12*, 12
skill development 137–138, *138*; switch 146–152, *147*, *150–152*
Smartbox: charities 187; communication boards 111–112; communication books 109; financial guidance 41; Grid software 60, *151–152*; symbol sets 59; training and support 40
SMART goals 163, 168
smoothie switches 144, *145*
SNUG (Spontaneous Novel Utterance Generation) 74
social model of disability 6
society, place in 179–180
speech generating devices *see* electronic AAC
spelling charts 117–118, *117*
static displays 14
Stepping Stones to Switch Access 148–149

stimming 70
structured lessons: modelling versus 85; teaching symbolic language 69, *70–71*
styli 139, *140*
SuperCore 14, *15*; AAC prompt hierarchy 125
switches 141–146, *144–147*
Switch Progression Road Map *147*, 148
switch scanning: and eye gaze technology 153; physical disabilities, learners with 143–146, *144–147*, 153–154
switch skill development 146–150, *147*, *150–152*
symbol charts *see* aided language displays
symbol generating software 45, 59, 62, 64, 103, 105; eye-pointing resources 114
symbolic hierarchy 23–25, *24*, 94
symbolic language: Communication Matrix 166; nature of 59–64; teaching 65–74
symbols, meaning of 10
symbol sets 13–14, *14*, 59–64; paper-based resources 105–106; teaching 65
SymbolStix *14*, 14, 62–64, *63*, 105; peer modelling case study 87
System for Augmented Language (SAL) 21

Talking Mats 177–178, *177–178*
target reviews: communication passports 35; teamwork 28–29, 34
target setting *see* assessment and target setting
T-bar stylus *140*
TD Snap Core First 14, *15*; vocabulary set 139, *139*
teaching symbolic language 65, 74; assigning meaning 65–68, *66–67*; babbling 70–72; communicative competencies 71–74; happy accidents 71; modelling 67–69; structured sessions 69, *70–72*
Teach Us Too 113
teamwork 27, 34; Affective Communication Assessment 99; communication passports 30–34, *31–32*; Education, Health and Care Plans 28–29; eye gaze technology 155; integrated therapy reviews 28–29; interventions 28–29, *29*; joint assessment process 27; joint target setting 27–28; modelling 85; physical disabilities, learners with 155; reviewing targets 28–29; *see also* multidisciplinary team
technical barriers 42
time barriers 42; communication partners 122
Tobii Dynavox: communication books 109; Dynamic AAC Goals Grid-3 164–165; eye gaze technology 154, *154*; symbol sets 59, 60, 61; training and support 40
Total Communication 1; environment 9
touch access 137–141, *138–141*
Touch Chat 14, *15*, 83
touch guides 141, *141*
touch pads 155–156, *155*
trackballs 156, *156*
training 38–43; AAC policy 185–186; modelling 85; Talking Mats 178
troubleshooting 42

unaided communication 10
United Nations (UN): Convention on the Rights of Persons with Disabilities 2; Convention on the Rights of the Child 2, 173
Universal Core Selection Tool 137

Van Oosterom, Judy 61
vision, school's 182, *183*
visual impairment 59, 61
visual scenes 14, *15*
vocabulary: meaning 14; modelling 78; organisation of 106; *see also* core vocabulary; fringe vocabulary
voice output communication aids *see* electronic AAC

whole school approach *see* AAC policy
Widgit symbols *14*, 14, 60–62, *62*, *63*, 64, 105; peer modelling case study 87; weather *82*
wired switches 144–146, *144–146*
wobble switches 144, *144*
word mats 50, *50*
WordPower 14, *15*

For Product Safety Concerns and Information please contact our EU
representative GPSR@taylorandfrancis.com
Taylor & Francis Verlag GmbH, Kaufingerstraße 24, 80331 München, Germany

www.ingramcontent.com/pod-product-compliance
Lightning Source LLC
Chambersburg PA
CBHW061539010526
44112CB00023B/2894